Peter Koch

Gesundheitliche Belastungen und Beanspruchungen von Erzieher/-innen

Peter Koch

Gesundheitliche Belastungen und Beanspruchungen von Erzieher/-innen

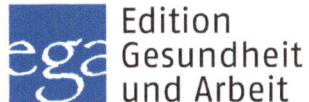

ega
Edition
Gesundheit
und Arbeit

© 2018
Edition Gesundheit und Arbeit,
Schriftenreihe des CVcare, Band 11
*Gesundheitliche Belastungen und Beanspruchungen
von Erzieher/-innen*

Universitätsklinikum Hamburg-Eppendorf (UKE),
CVcare | Bethanien-Höfe Eppendorf
Martinistraße 52, 20246 Hamburg
www.uke.de

Herausgeber
Prof. Dr. med. Albert Nienhaus
a.nienhaus@uke.de

Autor
Peter Koch

Redaktion
Elisabeth Muth

Gestaltung
Ethel Knop

Verlag
tredition GmbH, Hamburg
ISBN: 978-3-7439-9748-6

Bibliografische Information der Deutschen Nationalbibliothek
Die Deutsche Nationalbibliothek verzeichnet diese Publikation in der Deutschen Nationalbibliografie;
detaillierte bibliografische Daten sind im Internet über http://dnb.d-nb.de abrufbar.

Inhaltsverzeichnis

Vorwort Herausgeber

Die Edition Gesundheit und Arbeit (ega) ist eine Schriftenreihe des Competenzzentrums für Epidemiologie und Versorgungsforschung bei Pflegeberufen (CVcare) am Universitätsklinikum Hamburg-Eppendorf (UKE).

Mit der *ega* soll die Diskussion im deutschsprachigen Raum über effektive und effiziente Wege zur Verbesserung des Gesundheitsschutzes, der betrieblichen Gesundheitsförderung sowie des betrieblichen Gesundheitsmanagements unter besonderer Berücksichtigung der betrieblichen Wiedereingliederung sowie der Rehabilitation gefördert werden. Die *ega* ist eine Plattform für interdisziplinäre Beiträge aus der arbeitsweltbezogenen Gesundheitsforschung. Die Disziplinen Psychologie, Arbeitsmedizin, Gesundheitswissenschaften, Gesundheitsökonomie, Rehabilitations- und Versorgungsforschung sollen damit näher zusammengeführt und zum gegenseitigen Austausch angeregt werden.

Das CVcare ist Teil des Institutes für Versorgungsforschung in der Dermatologie und bei Pflegeberufen (IVDP) am UKE. Die Grundfinanzierung des CVcare wird durch eine Stiftung der Berufsgenossenschaft für Gesundheitsdienst und Wohlfahrtspflege (BGW) sichergestellt. Das CVcare kooperiert daher eng mit der BGW und hier insbesondere mit deren Forschungsbereich Grundlagen der Prävention und Rehabilitation (GPR).

Das CVcare stellt epidemiologische Daten zur Arbeits- und Gesundheitssituation von Pflegekräften und anderen Beschäftigten im Gesundheitswesen und in der Wohlfahrtspflege zur Verfügung. Angebote zur arbeitsweltbezogenen Gesundheitsförderung, Prävention und Rehabilitation werden unter besonderer Berücksichtigung des demografischen Wandels im Sinne der Versorgungsforschung überprüft. In praxisorientierten Projekten werden Vorschläge zur weiteren Verbesserung dieser Angebote entwickelt.

Schwerpunktthemen des CVcare sind die Arbeitssituation älterer Beschäftigter in der Pflege, arbeitsbedingte Beschwerden des Bewegungsapparates (MSB), Infektionsrisiken mit den Schwerpunkten Nadelstichverletzungen, Tuberkulose und multiresistente Erreger (MRE), psychosoziale Belastungen am Arbeitsplatz mit dem besonderen Schwerpunkt Gewalt am Arbeitsplatz sowie die Evaluation der Rehabilitationsleistungen der BGW und anderer Träger der gesetzlichen Unfallversicherung (GUV).

Der elfte Band der Edition gibt die Promotionsarbeit „Gesundheitliche Belastungen und Beanspruchungen von Erzieher/-innen" von Peter Koch wieder. Im Rahmen dieses Promotionsprojektes wurden Erzieher/-innen in einer Querschnitts- und in einer Längsschnittstudie zu Risikofaktoren für Beschwerden des Bewegungsapparates und Burnout befragt. Weiterhin wurde in einer Subgruppe die Wirksamkeit von persönlichem Gehörschutz (Otoplastiken) in Bezug auf Lärm und Burnout untersucht. Sowohl Beschwerden des Bewegungsapparates als auch Burnout-Symptome waren häufig. Ein wichtiger Risikofaktor war ein ungünstiges Verhältnis von Verausgabungen und Belohnungen (Effort-Reward-Imbalance). Allerdings konnten die Zusammenhänge aus der Querschnittsstudie nicht eindeutig in der Längsschnittstudie bestätigt werden. Die Studie zu den Otoplastiken (eine besondere Form von Gehörschutz, die Verständigung erlaubt) war von den Erzieher/-innen selber initiiert worden, mit dem Wunsch, diese Maßnahme zur Lärmreduktion auszuprobieren und wissenschaftlich evaluieren zu lassen. Bei den begleitenden raumakustischen Untersuchungen zeigte sich, dass die Raumakustik in den meisten Kindertagesstätten (Kita) nicht optimal war. Die Otoplastiken erwiesen sich nicht als geeignetes Mittel, die Lärmbelastung zu reduzieren, da sie im Laufe des Projektes immer seltener getragen wurden. Umso wichtiger erscheint es, technische und organisatorische Maßnahmen zur Reduktion der Lärmbelastung zu ergreifen. Das wird nicht nur den Erzieher/-innen sondern auch den Kindern zugutekommen.

Ich hatte die Freude, die Promotionsarbeit von Peter Koch zusammen mit Prof. Dr. Olaf von dem Knesebeck, Direktor des Instituts für Medizinische Soziologie am UKE, und Prof. Dr. Volker Harth, Leiter des Zentralinstitutes für Arbeitsmedizin und Schifffahrtsmedizin (ZfAM), Hamburg, zu betreuen. Für die Unterstützung und gute Zusammenarbeit möchte ich mich hier bei beiden bedanken.

Es freut mich, dem interessierten Leser die Arbeit zu Gesundheitlichen Belastungen und Beanspruchungen von Erzieher/-innen in der Schriftenreihe *ega* zur Verfügung stellen zu können.

Hamburg, im November 2018   Prof. Dr. med. Albert Nienhaus

Zusammenfassung

Einleitung

Bedingt durch den gesellschaftlichen Wunsch, Familie und Beruf besser zu vereinen, erfolgte in den vergangenen Jahren in Deutschland ein quantitativer und qualitativer Ausbau der Kindertagesstätten (Kitas). Demzufolge sind die Arbeitsbedingungen von Erzieher/-innen verstärkt in den Fokus geraten. Aktuelle Studien über Erzieher/-innen berichten über hohe Lärmbelastungen und ein ungünstiges Verhältnis von Anforderungen und Belohnungen (Effort-Reward-Imbalance (ERI)). In dieser Arbeit wurde ein Ausschnitt gesundheitlicher Beanspruchungen (muskuloskelettale Beschwerden (MSB) und Burnout) den Belastungen durch Effort-Reward-Imbalance gegenübergestellt sowie die Möglichkeit der Lärmprävention durch persönlichen Gehörschutz (Otoplastiken) bei Erzieher/-innen untersucht.

Methoden

In Studie 1 wurden bei Erzieher/-innen eines Trägers für Kinder- und Jugendeinrichtungen die Prävalenzen von ERI, MSB und Burnout im Querschnitt erhoben. Es wurde untersucht, in welcher Einrichtungsart die am höchsten belasteten Beschäftigten arbeiteten. In Studie 2 wurde der Einfluss von ERI auf MSB bzw. von ERI auf Burnout im Längsschnitt untersucht. Es sollte geprüft werden, inwiefern der ERI-Fragebogen als arbeitsmedizinisches Screening-Instrument für gesundheitliche Risikogruppen eingesetzt werden kann. Anhand einer Pilot-Interventionsstudie wurde in Studie 3 untersucht, ob der Einsatz von Otoplastiken die subjektive Lärmbelastung und das Burnout-Risiko bei Erzieher/-innen reduzieren kann.

Ergebnisse

Die Prävalenzen von ERI, Burnout und MSB lagen zum Zeitpunkt der Baseline-Untersuchung bei 65 %, 57 % bzw. bei 17 bis 59 %. Das Personal aus Kitas wies im Vergleich zu anderen Einrichtungsarten das höchste Belastungsprofil auf. Unter Berücksichtigung von körperlicher Belastung war ERI im Längsschnitt ein statistisch signifikanter Einflussfaktor für MSB (Kreuz: OR 4,2, Nacken: OR 4,3, MSB gesamt: OR 4,0). In Bezug auf Burnout zeigte sich bei einer Erhöhung des ERI-Quotienten um 10 % ein Anstieg des Burnout-Werts um 1,1 Punkte (95 %-CI: 0,09-2,14). Der Einsatz von Otoplastiken konnte die subjektive Lärmbelastung bzw. das Burnout nicht reduzieren, die Zufriedenheit mit den Geräten nahm über die Zeit ab. Bei über der Hälfte der Einrichtungen wurde bei der raumakustischen Begutachtung ein Verbesserungspotenzial festgestellt.

Fazit

Bei den Erzieher/-innen wurde eine hohe psychosoziale Belastung durch ein ungünstiges Verhältnis von Verausgabungen und Belohnungen beobachtet. Der ERI-Fragebogen eignet sich bei Erzieher/-innen als Screening-Instrument, um frühzeitig Risikogruppen in Bezug auf Burnout und MSB zu identifizieren. Die verhaltenspräventive Maßnahme zu Lärm zeigte im Arbeitsumfeld von Erzieher/-innen keinen Erfolg. Vielmehr sollten alle Maßnahmen auf der technisch-organisatorischen Ebene zur Optimierung der Raumakustik ausgeschöpft werden, um einen wirksamen Lärmschutz zu gewährleisten.

Abstract

Background

Due to the social desire for an improved reconciliation of work and family life, a quantitative and qualitative expansion of childcare has taken place in Germany in recent years. As a result the working conditions of child-care workers have come into public focus. Recent studies investigating childcare workers report on high noise exposures and an unfavorable balance of effort and reward (effort-reward imbalance). In this paper an excerpt of work-related strains (musculoskeletal symptoms and burnout) of childcare workers was related to the stress caused by effort-reward imbalance (ERI). Additionally an individual based noise-preventive measure for child-care workers (wearing moulded hearing protectors) was evaluated.

Methods

Study 1 investigated the prevalence rates of ERI, musculoskeletal symptoms (MS) and burnout in childcare workers of a funding provider for children and young people. It was also examined, in which type of institution the most stressed employees had worked. In study 2 the influence of effort-reward imbalance on MS and burnout respectively was tested with a longitudinal design. It should be investigated, if the ERI-questionnaire could be used as an occupational health screening instrument for identifying subgroups at a higher health risk. By means of an interventional pilot study, study 3 examined, whether the use of moulded hearing protectors (MHP's) could reduce subjective noise exposure and burnout risk in childcare workers.

Results

The baseline prevalence rates of effort-reward imbalance, burnout and MS were 65%, 57% and 17-59% respectively. The highest stresses and strains were observed for employees working in child day care centers in comparison to employees in other types of institutions. Based on the longitudinal data effort-reward imbalance was identified as a statistically significant predictor for MS, after adjusting especially for physical stress (lower back: OR 4.2, neck: OR 4.3, total MS: OR 4.0). With regard to burnout, a relative increase of 10% in the ERI ratio score increased the burnout score by 1.1 points (95% CI: 0.09-2.14). The application of MHP's could not reduce subjective noise exposure and burnout in childcare workers; the satisfaction of the study subjects with wearing MHP's decreased over time. An improvement of room acoustics was recommended for more than half of the institutions.

Conclusions

A high psychosocial stress by effort-reward imbalance has been observed for childcare workers. With regard to childcare workers the ERI questionnaire seems to be an eligible occupational health screening instrument for detecting subgroups that are at a higher risk to develop MS and burnout. Wearing MHP's as an individual based preventive measure showed no success in the work setting of childcare workers. In fact all measures on the technical and organizational level should be exploited to optimize the room acoustics in institutions of child care workers in order to perform occupational safety with respect to noise effectively.

Publikationsliste

P. Koch, J. Stranzinger, A. Nienhaus and A. Kozak (2015)

Musculoskeletal Symptoms and Risk of Burnout in Child Care Workers - A Cross-Sectional Study

PLoS One Oct 21;10(10):e0140980.

P. Koch, J. F. Kersten, J. Stranzinger and A. Nienhaus (2017)

The Effect of Effort-Reward Imbalance on the Health of Childcare Workers in Hamburg: A Longitudinal Study

Journal of Occupational Medicine and Toxicology Jun 26;12:16.

P. Koch, J. Stranzinger, J. F. Kersten and A. Nienhaus (2016)

Use of Moulded Hearing Protectors by Child Care Workers - An Interventional Pilot Study

Journal of Occupational Medicine and Toxicology Nov 8;11:50.

Synopse

1.1   Einleitung

Erzieher/-innen und Erzieher in Deutschland sind in den vergangenen Jahren stärker in das öffentliche Bewusstsein geraten: 2014 und 2015 kam es im kommunalen Sozial- und Erziehungsdienst zu bundesweiten Streiks. Die Erzieher/-innen forderten zur Anerkennung ihrer Arbeit eine Eingruppierung in eine höhere Entgeltgruppe und die Gewerkschaft ver.di kündigte die Eingruppierungsvorschriften (ver.di 2014).

Im Vorfeld dieser Streikwelle hatte das pädagogische Personal in Kitas wesentliche Veränderungen der strukturellen Rahmenbedingungen erfahren. Die Verabschiedung des „Gemeinsamen Rahmens der Länder für die frühe Bildung in Kindertageseinrichtungen" im Jahre 2004 führte zu einem neuen Qualifizierungsbedarf sowie zur Übernahme neuer Aufgaben (Jugendministerkonferenz 2004). Im Jahre 2013 trat zudem ein Gesetz in Kraft, das den rechtlichen Betreuungsanspruch für Kinder im Alter von ein bis unter drei Jahren regelte (SGB VIII 2008, § 24 Art. 1). Damit sollte die Verfügbarkeit von Kinderbetreuung ausgebaut werden, um die Vereinbarkeit von Familie und Beruf zu verbessern. Daten des Statistischen Bundesamts belegen, dass sich die Zahl der zu betreuenden Kinder in Kitas von 2006 bis 2016 um 15 % erhöht hat, von rund 2,9 auf 3,4 Millionen Kinder (Statistisches Bundesamt 2016). Parallel dazu wuchs auch die Zahl der pädagogisch tätigen Fachkräfte überproportional um 61 %, von rund 340.000 auf 550.000 Beschäftigte. Die Daten der amtlichen Statistik zeigen aber auch, dass sich der Anteil der Kinder, die eine Ganztagsbetreuung beanspruchen, in diesem Zeitraum relativ um 83 % erhöht (Abbildung 1) und der Anteil der betreuungsintensiven Kinder im Alter von null bis unter drei Jahren verdoppelt hat. Der positiven Entwicklung des Verhältnisses von pädagogisch Beschäftigten und betreuten Kindern in diesem Zeitraum steht eine relative Erhöhung der Arbeitslast in Kitas gegenüber. Angesichts der veränderten Rahmenbedingungen für die Arbeit in Kitas sowie der allgemeinen Überalterung der arbeitenden Bevölkerung, stellt sich die Frage, inwiefern Erzieher/-innen in Deutschland ihre Arbeitsbedingungen heutzutage als belastend empfinden und wie es um ihre Gesundheit bestellt ist. Da die Arbeit dieser Berufsgruppe die zentrale Stütze hinsichtlich des gesellschaftlichen Wunsches ist, Beruf und Familie besser zu vereinen, sollten die arbeitsbedingten Belastungen und die Gesundheit von Erzieher/-innen intensiver erforscht werden. Daraus folgende Erkenntnisse können eine gute Basis zur Entwicklung von betrieblichen Präventionsprogrammen zur Vermeidung von arbeitsbedingten Erkrankungen schaffen und/oder einen eventuellen Reformbedarf im Kita-Bereich aufzeigen. Untersuchungen belegen, dass strukturelle Rahmenbedingungen von Kitas nicht nur mit der Gesundheit und der Arbeitsfähigkeit von Erzieher/-innen in Zusammenhang stehen, sondern auch mit der pädagogischen Qualität, die einen Einfluss auf die Entwickungsverläufe der betreuten Kinder hat (Cryer 1999; Viernickel 2013).

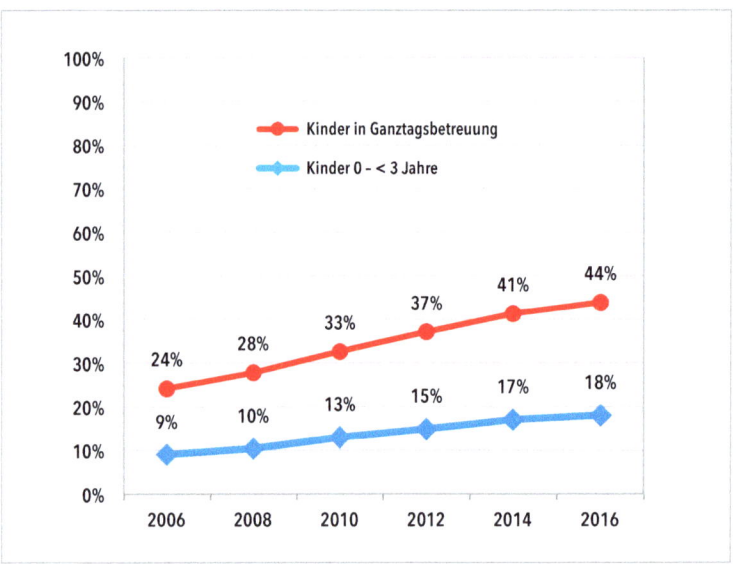

Abbildung 1 Anteile von betreuten Kinder in Kitas im Zeitverlauf (Statistisches Bundesamt 2016, eigene Berechnung)

1.2 Hintergrund

Aktuelle Untersuchungen zu deutschen Erzieher/-innen zeigen, dass die Arbeits-bedingungen durch Personalmangel, große Gruppen und Lärm dominiert wer-den (Fuchs-Rechlin 2007; Thinschmidt 2010, Krause-Girth 2011; Jungbauer 2015; Sinn-Behrendt 2015). Bei einer Erwerbstätigenbefragung des Bundesinstituts für Berufsbildung im Jahr 2012 lag die Lärmbelastung von Erzieher/-innen mit 55 % auf dem ersten Platz; dieser Anteil war fünfmal so hoch wie bei allen anderen Berufen (Hall 2015). Neben weiteren Untersuchungen, die die subjektive Lärmbelastung bei Erzieher/-innen bestätigen (Buch 2001; Schreyer 2014; Losch 2016), gibt es deutsche und internationale Studien, die anhand von Schalldruckpegelmessungen die erhöhte Lärmbelastungen für Erzieher/-innen objektiv erfassen (Buch 2001; Paulsen 2004; Eysel-Gosepath 2010; Sjodin 2012; Neitzel 2014; Sinn-Behrendt 2015). Die gemessenen Schalldruckspitzen liegen in diesen Studien über 85 dB(A) und damit über dem Schwellenwert von 80 dB(A), bei dessen Überschreitung der Arbeitgeber Maßnahmen zur Verhinderung bzw. Reduzierung des Lärms durchführen muss (LärmVibrationsArbSchV 2007). Weitere Belastungen, die in einer systematischen Übersichtsarbeit zu internationalen Studien aufgeführt werden, sind Arbeiten unter Zeitdruck, Multitasking, Konflikte mit Kollegen und Eltern, fehlende Anerkennung sowie das Empfinden einer unangemessenen Entlohnung für die Arbeit (McGrath 2007). Es gibt eine Reihe von deutschen Untersuchungen, die die psychosoziale Belastung dieser Berufsgruppe anhand des Verhältnisses von arbeitsbezogenen Verausgabungen und Belohnungen (ERI) erhoben haben (Siegrist 1996). In einer bundesweiten Repräsentativerhebung aus dem Jahr 2012 liegt der Anteil von Erzieher/-innen mit einem ungünstigen Verhältnis von Anforderungen und Belohnungen bei 67 % (ERI-Prävalenz), der entsprechende Mittelwert des ERI-Quotienten beträgt in dieser Studie 1,3 (Schreyer 2014). Eine weitere repräsentative Erhebung für Nordrhein-Westfalen aus dem Jahr 2010 beobachtete eine ERI-Prävalenz von 64 % bzw. einen Mittelwert des ERI-Quotienten von 1,3 (Viernickel 2013). Ältere Studien berichten von geringeren Ausprägungen; für 2007 wurde ein Mittelwert des ERI-Quotienten von 0,6 und für 2003 ein Mittelwert von 0,5 beobachtet (Scheuch 2007; Nübling 2013).

Als vorrangige Beanspruchungsfolgen in dieser Berufsgruppe werden in internationalen Übersichtsarbeiten unter anderem Burnout und MSB genannt (Bright 1999; McGrath 2007). Bei Erzieher/-innen in Deutschland werden Burnout-Raten zwischen zehn und 30 % beobachtet (Buch 2001; Rudow 2004; Jungbauer 2015). Burnout-Symptomatik bei Erzieher/-innen korreliert in Querschnittsstudien mit psychosozialen Faktoren wie geringem Handlungsspielraum und ERI (Scheuch 2007; Loerbroks 2014), Overcommitment (Nübling 2013), arbeitsbezogenen Konfliktsituationen und unangemessenem Gehalt (Goelman 1998), fehlender Anerkennung (Seti 2008) sowie mit Lärmbelastung (Sjodin 2012).

Aufgrund von Arbeiten in niedrigen Höhen und dem Heben und Tragen von Kindern sind bei deutschen Erzieher/-innen ebenfalls erhöhte MSB-Raten zu beobachten (BAUA 2016). In deutschen Studien werden für Erzieher/-innen Prävalenzen von Kreuzschmerzen (35 bis 65 %), Nackenschmerzen (16 bis 42 %), Schulterschmerzen (42 %) und allgemeine MSB (59 %) beschrieben (Rudow 2005; Viernickel 2013;

Hall 2015; Rudow 2015; Sinn-Behrendt 2015). Neben dem Einfluss der Biomechanik gibt es bei der Entstehung von arbeitsbedingten MSB auch Hinweise auf beteiligte psychosoziale Faktoren (Hoogendoorn 2000; Lang 2012; Kraatz 2013). Dies ist insbesondere bei schlecht bezahlten Berufsgruppen zu beobachten (Lundberg 1999). Der Zusammenhang zwischen dem Auftreten von MSB und den Faktoren des ERI-Modells ist bei Beschäftigungskollektiven aus anderen Branchen (Busfahrer, Callcenter-Beschäftigte, öffentliche Verwaltung) in Längsschnittstudien festgestellt worden (Rugulies 2008; Krause 2010; Lapointe 2013). In einem systematischen Review über alle Branchen wird der Zusammenhang von ERI und MSB anhand von Quer- und Längsschnittstudien allerdings als inkonsistent bewertet (Koch 2014).

Das Effort-Reward-Imbalance-Modell

Das ERI-Modell (Modell der beruflichen Gratifikationskrise) nach Siegrist erfasst die arbeitsbedingte psychosoziale Situation anhand eines Fragebogens (Siegrist 1996). Das Modell basiert auf der Annahme, dass geleistete Arbeit im Idealfall in wechselseitiger Beziehung zu gesellschaftlich definierten Belohnungen steht (Reziprozität). Die Gesundheit des Arbeitnehmers wird in Beziehung zu erbrachter Leistung und gewährten Belohnungen (Gehalt, Anerkennung, sicherer Arbeitsplatz und Aufstiegschancen) gesetzt (Abbildung 2). Liegt ein Ungleichgewicht von hoher Leistung und niedriger Belohnung vor, entsteht nach Siegrist eine Stresssituation, die bei anhaltender Dauer das Risiko für stressassoziierte Erkrankungen wie z.B. koronare Herzerkrankung, kardiovaskuläre Erkrankungen oder Depressionen erhöht (Siegrist 2008). Eine Besonderheit des ERI-Modells ist das Einbeziehen einer persönlichen Coping-Strategie bei hohen Arbeitsanforderungen: Overcommitment (OVC) ist ein exzessives Motivationsmuster, das eine hohe Leistungsbereitschaft bei einer hohen Belohnungserwartung erzeugt. Nach Siegrist haben Beschäftigte mit diesem Muster, die sich in einer beruflichen Gratifikationskrise befinden, ein noch höheres Erkrankungsrisiko als Beschäftigte ohne OVC. Der ERI-Quotient wird anhand einer Verhältnisformel aus den Verausgabungs- und Belohnungsskalenwerten berechnet, die die unterschiedliche Anzahl von Items der Skalen berücksichtigt. Eine ERI liegt vor, sobald der ERI-Quotient über dem Wert 1 liegt. Der Cut-off-Wert von OVC liegt verteilungsabhängig bei dem dritten Tertil der beobachteten Werte. Auf die detaillierte Beschreibung der Berechnungen des ERI-Quotienten und des OVC-Wertes soll hier nicht weiter eingegangen werden, sie sind der Originalliteratur zu entnehmen (Siegrist 2004).

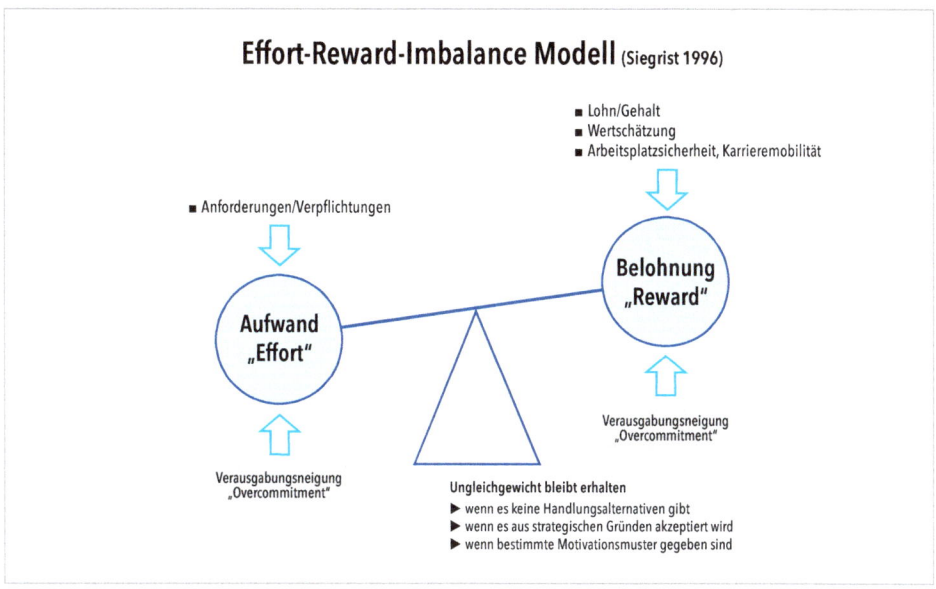

Abbildung 2 Komponenten des Effort-Reward-Imbalance-Modells (Siegrist 1996)

Der ERI-Fragebogen wurde bereits in einigen Untersuchungen zu den Arbeitsbedingungen bei deutschen Erzieher/-innen eingesetzt (Seibt 2006; Scheuch 2007; Nübling 2013; Viernickel 2013; Schreyer 2014). Der Vorteil, auf der Basis eines bekannten theoretischen Stressmodells psychosoziale Faktoren zu erheben, besteht zum einen darin, dass dazu eine Reihe von Vergleichsdaten vorliegt. Zum anderen können anhand der zugrundeliegenden Theorie der Stressentstehung gezielter präventive Maßnahmen formuliert und deren Effektivität evaluiert werden (Theorell 1999).

Die folgende Arbeit untersucht mit Methoden der Feldforschung gesundheitliche Belastungen und Beanspruchungen von deutschen Erzieher/-innen sowie die Möglichkeit der Lärmprävention. Sie beschäftigt sich nicht mit allen Belastungen und Beanspruchungen, sondern legt den Focus auf Lärm, ERI, Burnout und MSB.

Den ursprünglichen Impuls für diese Untersuchungen gaben die Beschäftigten eines Hamburger Trägers für Kinder- und Jugendeinrichtungen selbst: Aufgrund von Lärmbelastung fingen Erzieher/-innen eigeninitiativ an, während der Arbeit Otoplastiken (persönlichen Gehörschutz) zu tragen. In Zusammenarbeit mit Geschäftsführung, Betriebsrat, Betriebsarzt und der Berufsgenossenschaft für Gesundheitsdienst und Wohlfahrtspflege wurde in diesem Kontext eine Maßnahme zur Lärmprävention entwickelt und durchgeführt. Parallel fanden im Abstand von einem Jahr zwei Mitarbeiterbefragungen statt, mit denen die psychosozialen Belastungen und die gesundheitlichen Beanspruchungen der Beschäftigten erhoben wurden.

Diese Arbeit setzt sich aus drei Veröffentlichungen zusammen, die im Rahmen des PhD-Programms für Nichtmediziner/-innen am Universitätsklinikum Hamburg-Eppendorf (UKE) entstanden sind. Die erste Publikation beschreibt die Ergebnisse der ersten Mitarbeiterbefragung (Querschnittsstudie). In dieser Publikation wurden ERI und weitere arbeitsbezogene Belastungen und Ressourcen sowie die Prävalenzen von Burnout und MSB bei den beschäftigten Erzieher/-innen in den verschiedenen Einrichtungen sowie der Einfluss von ERI auf Burnout bzw. MSB dargestellt. Im Kontext einer betrieblichen Gefährdungsbeurteilung dienten diese Informationen zur Entwicklung von präventiven Maßnahmen.

In der zweiten Publikation wurden die Daten der ersten und zweiten Mitarbeiterbefragung im Längsschnitt untersucht (Kohortenstudie). Hier wurde der zeitliche Verlauf der ERI-, Burnout- und MSB-Prävalenzen dargestellt. Weiterhin wurde untersucht, inwiefern ERI Einfluss auf eine Erhöhung der Burnout- bzw. MSB-Prävalenzen im Längsschnitt hat. Bei einem Nachweis eines potenziellen statistisch signifikanten Zusammenhangs zwischen den Faktoren des ERI-Modells und MSB bzw. Burnout könnte der ERI-Fragebogen aus arbeitsmedizinischer Sicht mehr Bedeutung für die Prävention gewinnen: Beschäftigte mit ERI würden als eine MSB-und/oder Burnout-Risikogruppe identifiziert werden können und präventive Maßnahmen könnten somit frühzeitig und gezielt durchgeführt werden.

Die dritte Publikation beschreibt die Ergebnisse der betrieblichen Präventionsmaßnahme zu Lärm (Otoplastikenstudie). Hier wurden die Nutzungszufriedenheit mit den Otoplastiken und die Effektivität in Bezug auf die Reduktion subjektiver Lärmbelastung und Burnout untersucht. Zusätzlich erfolgte eine raumakustische Begutachtung der Einrichtungen, in denen die Studienteilnehmer/-innen beschäftigt waren. Anhand der Ergebnisse dieser Studie sollte ein Fazit gezogen werden, ob das Tragen von Otoplastiken als Maßnahme der Verhaltensprävention bei Erzieher/-innen als geeignet und sinnvoll zu bewerten ist.

Da in Querschnittsstudien die zeitliche Chronologie zwischen Exposition und Outcome nicht nachvollziehbar ist, kann keine Aussage über die ätiologische Beziehung von Krankheitsursache und Krankheit getroffen werden (Gordis 2001, S.183). Aus diesem Grund wurden in der Mantelarbeit Assoziationen nur auf der Grundlage der Längsschnittdaten angegeben (Kohortenstudie), auf die Präsentation der Assoziationsmaße aus der Querschnittsstudie wurde somit verzichtet.

Die Teilnehmer/-innen in den drei Studien überlappen sich teilweise. Zu beachten ist, dass die Proband/-innen der Otoplastikenstudie eine Subgruppe der Teilnehmer/-innen der Kohortenstudie sind und diese beiden Studien zeitlich parallel verlaufen (Abbildung 3).

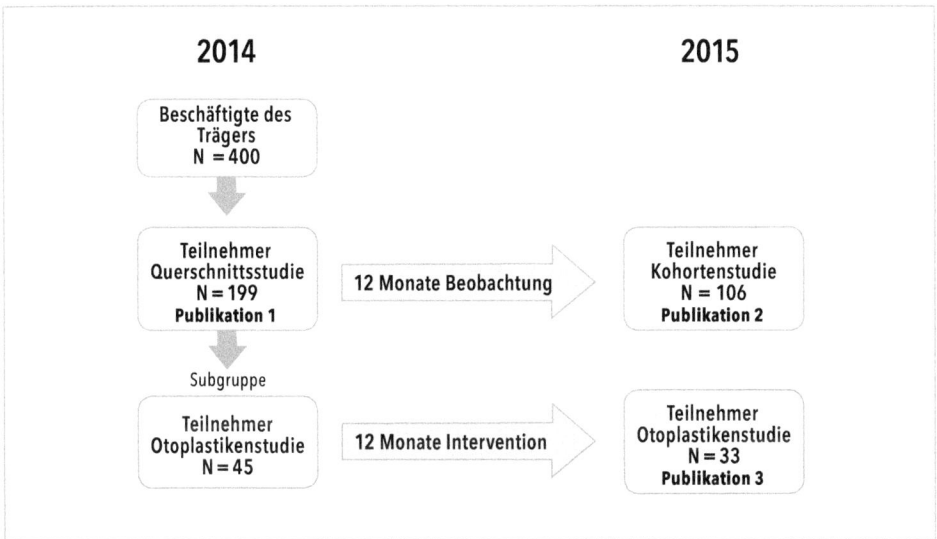

Abbildung 3 Rekrutierung der Studienteilnehmer/-innen

Beschäftigte in Kindertagesstätten, Horten und anderen pädagogischen Einrichtungen für Kinder und Jugendliche können verschiedene Fachausbildungen haben, z.B. Ausbildungen zu Erzieher/-innen, Heilpädagog/-innen, Heilerziehungspfleger/-innen, sozialpädagogischen Assistent/-innen, Sozialpädagog/-innen. Da in den vorliegenden Untersuchungen die Fachqualifikation nicht erhoben worden ist, bezieht sich der Begriff „Erzieher/-innen" auf alle Beschäftigten, die im weiteren Sinne eine pädagogische Ausbildung haben und pädagogisch tätig sind.

Alle drei Studien wurden mit dem Datenschutzbeauftragten des Trägers sowie mit der Ethikkommission der Hamburger Ärztekammer abgestimmt.

1.3 Studie 1 – Musculoskeletal Symptoms and Risk of Burnout in Child Care Workers (Querschnittsstudie)

1.3.1 Studienziel

Im Rahmen einer betrieblichen Gefährdungsbeurteilung sollten anhand der ersten Mitarbeiterbefragung im Jahr 2014 die subjektiv wahrgenommenen Belastungen, Ressourcen und Beanspruchungsfolgen der Erzieher/-innen in den verschiedenen Einrichtungstypen des Trägers ermittelt werden. Folgende Einrichtungstypen wurden von dem Träger für Kinder und Jugendeinrichtungen betrieben: In Kitas werden Kinder im Alter bis zu sechs Jahren, in sogenannten Schulkooperationen Schulkinder an Ganztagsschulen in der unterrichtsfreien Nachmittagszeit betreut und bei den Einrichtungen der Kinder- und Jugendförderung handelt es sich um Wohngruppen und Jugendprojekte, in denen ebenfalls Kinder im Schulalter betreut werden. Folgende Forschungsfrage sollte anhand der Studie beantwortet werden: Wie hoch sind die arbeitsbedingten Belastungen und Ressourcen sowie die MSB- und Burnout-Prävalenzen bei den Erzieher/-innen in den verschiedenen Einrichtungstypen des Trägers?

1.3.2 Methoden

Mit Unterstützung des Betriebsrats wurde der Fragebogen an 400 Beschäftigte in 26 verschiedenen Einrichtungen des Trägers verteilt. Mit Ausblick auf ein späteres Follow-up wurde die Befragung in pseudonymisierter Form durchgeführt. Eingeschlossen wurden alle Beschäftigten, die eine Mindestarbeitszeit von zehn Stunden in der Woche angegeben hatten und im pädagogischen Bereich oder/und dessen Leitung tätig waren.
Neben demografischen Informationen umfasste der Fragebogen Angaben zu berufsbezogenen Belastungen und Ressourcen, als Outcomes wurden Burnout und MSB erhoben (Abbildung 4).

Insgesamt beteiligten sich 230 Beschäftigte an der Befragung (Response-Rate: 57 %). 31 Beschäftigte mit einer zu geringen Arbeitszeit bzw., die nicht pädagogisch tätig waren, wurden aus der Analyse ausgeschlossen.

Statistische Analyse

Für Gruppenvergleiche von kategorialen Daten wurde der Chi²-Test einge-
setzt. Für Gruppenvergleiche von normalverteilten Daten wurden einfaktorielle
Varianzanalysen durchgeführt. Bei begründeter Annahme der Verletzung der
Normalverteilungsvoraussetzung wurde das nicht parametrische Äquivalent, der
Kruskal-Wallis-Test, eingesetzt. Das Signifikanzniveau lag bei $p < 0,05$. Die Aus-
wertung erfolgte mit dem Statistikpaket SPSS-Version 22.

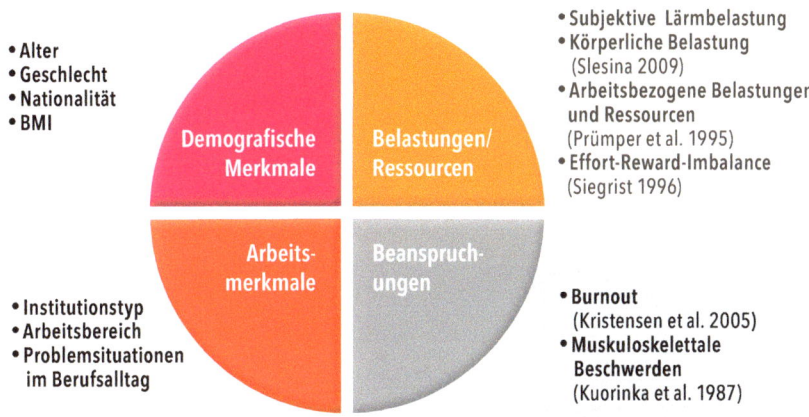

Abbildung 4 Inhalte des Fragebogens der Mitarbeiterbefragung

1.3.3 Ergebnisse

Insgesamt gingen die Daten von 199 Erzieher/-innen in die Analyse ein. Die Teil-
nehmer/-innen der Befragung waren überwiegend Frauen (86 %). Die stärkste
Altersgruppe waren die 40- bis 50-Jährigen (29 %), das Durchschnittsalter lag bei
40 Jahren. Über 90 % besaßen die deutsche Staatsangehörigkeit. Von den Teil-
nehmer/-innen kamen 56 % aus Kindertagesstätten, 26 % arbeiteten in Schulkooperationen und ein geringer Teil (10 %) kam aus Einrichtungen der Kinder- und
Jugendförderung.

Die Mittelwerte der Ressourcen Handlungsspielraum ($\bar{x}$: 3,7), Vielseitigkeit ($\bar{x}$: 3,8),
Ganzheitlichkeit ($\bar{x}$: 3,7), Information und Mitsprache ($\bar{x}$: 3,8) sowie Zusammenarbeit ($\bar{x}$: 3,7) lagen für die Gesamtgruppe im Bereich von ca. 75 % der höchst-
möglichen Ausprägung (Wertebereich 1–5). Die Beschäftigten in den Einrichtungen der Kinder-und Jugendförderung wiesen dabei die höchsten Mittelwerte auf.

Bezüglich der Problemsituationen beschrieb ein großer Teil der Teilnehmer/
-innen (89 %) die Situation bei der Arbeit als zu laut (Tabelle 1). Am häufigsten traf
dies bei den Beschäftigten der Kitas (94 %) zu. Am zweithäufigsten wurde eine
zu große Gruppenstärke genannt (78 %). Über die Hälfte der Befragten gab an,
regelmäßig Konflikte mit Eltern zu haben (58 %), am geringsten betraf dies die
Beschäftigten aus der Kinder-und Jugendförderung (38 %). Konflikte mit Kollegen
wurden am häufigsten von Beschäftigten aus den Kitas genannt (60 %). Fehlende
Pausen gaben 50 % und Konflikte mit der Leitung 32 % der Teilnehmer/-innen
an. Mit schreienden und schwer beeinflussbaren Kindern hatten am häufigsten
Beschäftigte der Kitas zu tun (80 %).

Tabelle 1 Beschreibung der Problemsituationen im Berufsalltag nach Einrichtungsarten (N = 186)

Problemsituationen	Kitas (n = 112)	Schulkoope-rationen (n = 53)	Kinder- u. Jugend-förderung (n = 21)	Gesamt (n = 186)
	Anteil (n)	Anteil (n)	Anteil (n)	Anteil (n)
Bei meiner Arbeit ist es oft zu laut.*	94 % (105)	87 % (46)	67 % (14)	89 % (165)
Unsere Gruppenstärken sind zu groß.	79 % (85)	80 % (41)	60 % (12)	78 % (138)
Es gibt Konflikte mit Eltern.	61 % (68)	60 % (32)	38 % (8)	58 % (108)
Es gibt Konflikte mit Kollegen.*	60 % (67)	42 % (22)	29 % (6)	51 % (95)
Es fehlen Pausen.	43 % (47)	60 % (32)	62 % (13)	50 % (92)
Es gibt Konflikte mit der Leitung.	36 % (39)	23 % (12)	33 % (7)	32 % (58)
Es gibt Kinder, die plötzlich losschreien und nicht beeinflusst werden können.	80 % (86)	72 % (38)	57 % (12)	75 % (136)

*p < 0,01

Hinsichtlich der körperlichen Belastung und der subjektiven Lärmbelastung wurden bei den Beschäftigten in den Kitas die höchsten Ausprägungen beobachtet. Bei
beiden Belastungsvariablen waren die Unterschiede zwischen den Beschäftigten
der drei Einrichtungsarten statistisch signifikant (p < 0,001).

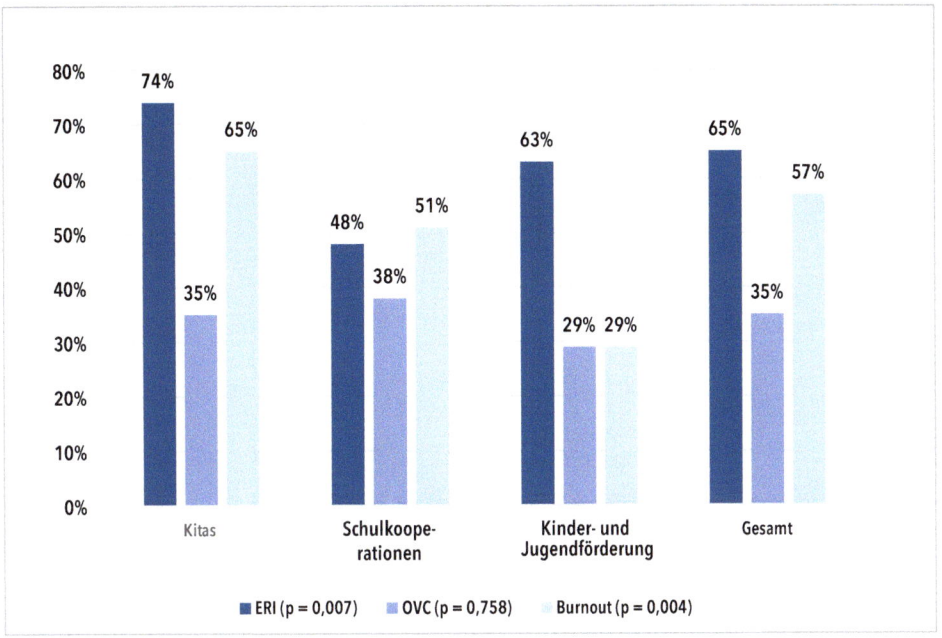

Abbildung 5 Verteilung von Effort-Reward-Imbalance, OVC und Burnout über die Institutionsarten

Für die Gesamtgruppe wurde eine ERI-Prävalenz von 65 % beobachtet ($\bar{x}$: 1,17; SD: 0,37), bei 35 % der Teilnehmer/innen lag ein OVC vor (Cut-off-Wert 3.Tertil: 16,6) (Abbildung 5). Die Kita-Beschäftigten wiesen die höchste ERI-Prävalenz auf (74 %), dieser Unterschied zwischen den verschiedenen Einrichtungsarten war statistisch signifikant. Bei der Mehrheit der Stichprobe (57 %) wurde ein Burnout festgestellt ($\bar{x}$: 51,7; SD: 18,2). Mit 65 % war die Burnout-Prävalenz bei den Kita-Beschäftigten am höchsten ($\bar{x}$: 54,8; SD: 18,3), auch dieser Unterschied zwischen den Einrichtungsarten war statistisch signifikant.

Tabelle 2 beschreibt die Prävalenzen von chronischen MSB. Kreuzschmerzen wurden mit 40 % am häufigsten angegeben, die Prävalenzen von Nackenschmerzen und Schulterschmerzen lagen bei 35 % bzw. 16 %. Das Vorliegen von mindestens einer der drei Schmerzlokalisationen (MSB gesamt) traf bei 59 % der Teilnehmer/-innen zu. Im Gruppenvergleich waren die höchsten Prävalenzen für Kreuz-, Schulterschmerzen und MSB gesamt bei den Beschäftigten der Kitas (46 %, 17 % und 62 %), der höchste Anteil für Nackenschmerzen bei Beschäftigten der Schulkooperationen zu beobachten (48 %).

Tabelle 2 Häufigkeiten von MSB bei Beschäftigten in den verschiedenen Einrichtungsarten (N = 186)

	Kitas (n = 112)	Schulkoope-rationen (n = 53)	Kinder- u. Jugend-förderung (n = 21)	Gesamt (n = 186)	
	Anteil	Anteil	Anteil	Anteil	p
Schulter (fehlende Werte n = 18)	17%	15%	11%	16%	0,733
Nacken (fehlende Werte n = 23)	31%	48%	25%	35%	0,061
Kreuz (fehlende Werte n = 22)	46%	33%	22%	40%	0,081
MSB gesamt (fehlende Werte n = 30)	62%	56%	47%	59%	0,454

1.3.4 Diskussion

Im Rahmen einer betrieblichen Gefährdungsbeurteilung liefert die Befragung Daten zu den arbeitsbezogenen Belastungen, Ressourcen und Beanspruchungen der Beschäftigten in den verschiedenen Einrichtungsarten. Die Ergebnisse der Studie zeigen, dass in dieser Stichprobe von Erzieher/-innen mit einer Prävalenz von 57% ($\bar{x}$ = 54,8) ein erhebliches Burnout-Risiko vorliegt. Daten aus Vergleichsstudien ermittelten Prävalenzen von 10 bis 30% (Buch 2001; Rudow 2004; Jungbauer 2015), der Mittelwert der Referenzdaten bei Erzieher/-innen der Copenhagen Psychosocial Questionnaire (COPSOQ)-Datenbank aus dem Jahr 2013 liegt mit 48 unter dem beobachteten Wert von 51,7 (Nübling 2015). Die beobachteten Prävalenzen von MSB (Schulter: 17%, Nacken: 35%, Kreuz: 40% und MSB gesamt: 59%) liegen nicht höher bzw. entsprechen den Anteilswerten von MSB aus anderen Studien bei Erzieher/-innen (Schulterschmerzen: 42% (Rudow 2015; Sinn-Behrendt 2015), Nackenschmerzen: 16 bis 42% (Rudow 2005; Rudow 2015; Sinn-Behrendt 2015), Kreuzschmerzen: 35 bis 65% (Rudow 2005; Hall 2015; Rudow 2015) und MSB gesamt: 59% (Viernickel 2013; Hall 2015; Rudow 2015). Die Prävalenz von Kreuzschmerzen ist verglichen mit der Prävalenz bei Beschäftigten aller anderen Berufen (46%) geringfügig niedriger, wie aus einer Erwerbstätigenbefragung hervorgeht (Hall 2015). Die ERI-Prävalenz von 65% bzw. der Mittelwert des ERI-Quotienten von 1,17 liegt im Bereich der beobachteten Werte aus den aktuellsten

Vergleichsstudien (Viernickel 2013, Schreyer 2014). Im Vergleich zu älteren Studien hebt sich der Mittelwert des ERI-Quotienten allerdings deutlich ab ($\bar{x}$ = 0,5, $\bar{x}$ = 0,6) (Scheuch 2007; Nübling 2013). Ebenso ist der Anteil von Beschäftigten mit OVC (35 %) vergleichbar mit dem Anteil (39 %) unter Erzieher/-innen aus einer aktuellen Auswertung des Sozio-oekonomischen Panels (SOEP) (Spieß 2016). Die trotz des hohen Belastungspotenzials positiv ausgeprägten Ressourcen wurden auch in weiteren Studien bei Erzieher/-innen beobachtet. In diesen Studien werden ähnlich hohe Werte z. B. in Bezug auf Vielseitigkeit, Handlungsspielraum, Information und Mitsprache genannt (Berger 2002; Rudow 2005; Fuchs 2008).

Die Ergebnisse der vorliegenden Querschnittsstudie verdeutlichen, dass sich insbesondere die Erzieher/-innen aus den Kitas durch ein erhöhtes Belastungs- (Lärm, Konflikte mit Eltern/Kollegen/Leitung, schwer beeinflussbare Kinder, ERI: 74 %) und ein erhöhtes Beanspruchungsprofil (MSB gesamt: 62 %, Burnout: 65 %) als Risikogruppe auszeichnen.

1.4 Studie 2 – The Effect of Effort-Reward Imbalance on the Health of Childcare Workers in Hamburg: A Longitudinal Study (Kohortenstudie)

1.4.1 Studienziel

Die Prävalenz von ERI bei deutschen Erzieher/-innen liegt nach aktuellen Schätzungen zwischen 64 % und 67 % und hat sich im Verlauf der vergangenen zehn Jahre deutlich erhöht (Viernickel 2013; Schreyer 2014; Koch 2015). In internationalen Studien wird bei Erzieher/-innen ein erhöhtes Risiko für MSB beobachtet (Bright 1999; McGrath 2007), der Zusammenhang zwischen ERI und MSB gilt als inkonsistent (Koch 2014). Längsschnittuntersuchungen zu diesem Zusammenhang sind rar, für die Berufsgruppe von Erzieher/-innen ist bislang dazu keine Studie publiziert worden. Ein erhöhtes Burnout-Risiko ist insbesondere bei Beschäftigten aus dem Dienstleistungssektor zu beobachten (Schaufeli 2003). Für deutsche Erzieher/-innen werden Prävalenzraten der Burnout-Symptomatik zwischen 10 % und 57 % angegeben (Buch 2001; Rudow 2004; Jungbauer 2015; Koch 2015). In Querschnittsstudien korreliert Burnout bei Erzieher/-innen und LehrerInnen stark mit ERI bzw. OVC (Scheuch 2007; Koch 2015) sowie branchenübergreifend mit OVC (Nübling 2013). Längsschnittuntersuchungen zu dem Zusammenhang von ERI und Burnout bei Erzieher/-innen sind bislang nicht publiziert worden.

Eine Untersuchung zu dem Zusammenhang von ERI und Burnout bzw. ERI und MSB ist aus arbeitsmedizinischer Sicht relevant, da bei einem bestehenden Zusammenhang der Einsatz des ERI-Fragebogens ein präventives Potenzial erschließen würde: Psychosozial belastete Beschäftigte könnten vor dem Eintreten von Beanspruchungsfolgen frühzeitig identifiziert und es könnten gezielt präventive Maßnahmen eingeleitet werden.

Folgende Forschungsfragen sollten in dieser Untersuchung beantwortet werden:

1. Zeigt sich bei Erzieher/-innen im Längsschnitt ein Zusammenhang zwischen den psychosozialen Faktoren des ERI-Modells und dem Auftreten von MSB?
2. Zeigt sich bei Erzieher/-innen im Längsschnitt ein Zusammenhang zwischen den psychosozialen Faktoren des ERI-Modells und einem erhöhten Burnout-Risiko?

1.4.2 Methoden

In der Kohortenstudie wurden die Teilnehmer/innen der Querschnittsstudie (Studie 1) über zwölf Monate weiterverfolgt. Zum Zeitpunkt des Follow-up wurde der Fragebogen der Querschnittsuntersuchung eingesetzt, d.h. es wurden erneut Daten zu den arbeitsbezogenen Belastungen und Ressourcen, ERI, Burnout und MSB erhoben (siehe Kapitel 1.3.2).

Statistische Analyse:

Hinsichtlich der ersten in Abschnitt 1.4.1 genannten Fragestellung wurden schrittweise multivariate logistische Regressionsmodelle gerechnet. Beginnend mit einem Kernvariablenset (ERI, körperliche Belastung, MSB zu T_0, Teilnahme an Otoplastikenstudie) wurden sämtliche Variablen ins Modell aufgenommen, die in der bivariaten Auswertung einen p-Wert <0,25 aufwiesen (Hosmer and Lemeshow 2000). Bezüglich der zweiten in Abschnitt 1.4.1 genannten Fragestellung wurde im linearen Regressionsmodell ebenfalls von einem Kernvariablenset ausgegangen (ERI, Burnout zu T_0, Alter, Teilnahme an Otoplastikenstudie, Einrichtungsart). Im ersten Schritt wurden ebenfalls sämtliche Variablen eingeschlossen, die in der bivariaten Auswertung einen p-Wert von <0,25 aufwiesen. Im zweiten Schritt wurde die Stepwise-backwards-Prozedur angewandt (Hosmer and Lemeshow 2000), wobei die Variablen mit einem p-Wert >0,1 aus dem Modell ausgeschlossen wurden. Um die Voraussetzung symmetrischer Residuen für die Anwendung der linearen Regression zu erfüllen, wurde die ERI-Variable vor den Berechnungen logarithmiert. In allen multivariaten Analysen ist eine potenzielle Interaktion von ERI und OVC überprüft worden. Eine Drop-out-Analyse wurde mittels logistischer Regression durchgeführt. Die statistische Auswertung erfolgte mit SPSS Statistics, Version 23.

1.4.3 Ergebnisse

Zum Zeitpunkt des Follow-up umfasste die Kohorte 106 Beschäftigte (Follow-up-Rate: 53%), 91% davon waren Frauen (Tabelle 3). Mehr als 90% besaßen die deutsche Staatsbürgerschaft. Knapp 53% waren in Vollzeit beschäftigt, 66% arbeiteten in Kitas, 22% in Schulkooperationen und 11% in Einrichtungen der Kinder- und Jugendförderungen. Die Studienteilnehmer/-innen im Follow-up waren im Mittel statistisch signifikant älter als die Drop-outs (43 vs. 37 Jahre, p <0,001), das Alter war die einzig statistisch signifikante Variable in der Drop-out-Analyse.

Über die Beobachtungszeit erhöhte sich der Mittelwert des ERI-Quotienten von 1,2 (SD: 0,4) auf 1,3 (SD: 0,3) sowie der Anteil derjenigen mit einem ERI-Quotienten >1 von 65,1% auf 87,4%. Die Erhöhung sowohl in der kontinuierlichen als auch in der dichotomen ERI-Variable waren statistisch signifikant (p <0,001). Welche der ERI-Subskalen maßgeblich für den signifikanten Anstieg des ERI-Quotienten verantwortlich ist, ist in Abbildung 6 ersichtlich.

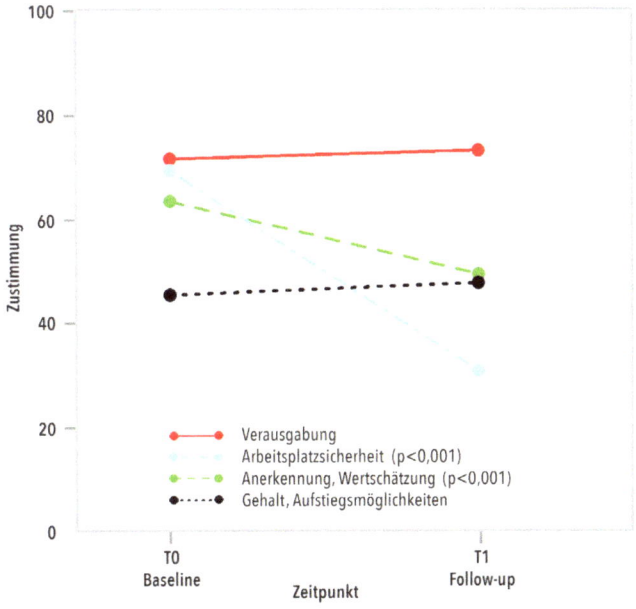

Abbildung 6 Mittelwerte der ERI-Belohnungssubskalen auf normierter 100er-Skala

Tabelle 3 Beschreibung der Kohorte zum Zeitpunkt des Follow-up

Variable	N	Prozent
Geschlecht		
Frauen	96	91%
Männer	10	9%
Alter in Jahren		
18–29	16	15%
30–39	22	21%
40–49	38	36%
50+	29	27%
fehlend	1	1%
Nationalität		
deutsch	98	92%
andere	8	8%
Wochenarbeitszeit		
Vollzeit	56	53%
Teilzeit	50	47%
Institution		
Kindertagesstätte	70	66%
Schulkooperation	23	22%
Kinder- und Jugendförderung	12	11%
fehlend	1	1%
Gesamt	**106**	**100%**

Der normierte Mittelwert der Skala *Verausgabung* war nahezu konstant geblieben (73 vs. 72). Für die drei Subskalen der Belohnungsskala war Folgendes zu beobachten: *Gehalt/Aufstiegsmöglichkeiten* nahm über die Zeit um 3 Punkte zu (45 vs. 48), *Anerkennung/Wertschätzung* und *Arbeitsplatzsicherheit* dagegen nahmen über die Zeit statistisch signifikant ab. Hier fiel der normierte Mittelwert von 62 auf 49 ($p < 0{,}001$) bzw. von 67 auf 31 Punkte ($p < 0{,}001$).

Die Ergebnisse der multivariaten logistischen Regression (Tabelle 4) zeigten für das Outcome Kreuzschmerzen ein statistisch signifikantes Odds Ratio von 4,2 für Personen mit einem ERI-Quotienten >1 (95%-CI: 1,14-15,50, $p = 0{,}031$). Für Schulterschmerzen war bei einem ERI-Quotienten >1 ein Odds Ratio von 1,5 (95 %-CI: 0,40-5,58) zu beobachten, das statistisch nicht signifikant war. In Bezug auf Nackenschmerzen wurde bei einem ERI-Quotienten >1 ein statistisch signifikantes Odds Ratio von 4,3 ermittelt (95 %-CI: 1,25–15,0, p = 0,021). Bei dem Outcome MSB gesamt ergab sich für Beschäftigte mit einem erhöhten ERI-Quotienten ebenfalls eine statistisch signifikante Erhöhung des Odds Ratio (OR: 4,0, 95 %-CI: 1,20-13,49, p = 0,024). Bei Beschäftigten, die angaben, Konflikte mit Eltern zu haben, zeigte sich ein statistisch signifikant erhöhtes Odds Ratio für eine Zunahme von MSB gesamt (OR: 4,9, 95 %-CI: 1,55-15,75, p = 0,007) (nicht aus Tabelle ersichtlich).

Bei Personen, die angaben, regelmäßig Sport zu treiben, zeigte sich ein statistisch signifikanter protektiver Effekt in Bezug auf das Auftreten von MSB (OR: 0,3, 95 %-CI: 0,10-0,98, p = 0,046) (nicht aus Tabelle ersichtlich). Eine Interaktion von ERI und OVC war in keinem der Modelle zu beobachten.

Tabelle 4 Ergebnisse der multivariaten logistischen Regressionen für MSB in den verschiedenen Körperregionen

	Kreuz[1] 35 % (36)			Schulter[2] 19 % (20)			Nacken[3] 39 % (41)			MSB gesamt[4] 62 % (64)		
	OR	95 %-CI	p	OR	95 %-CI	p	OR	95 %-CI	p	OR	95 %-CI	p
ERI >1 vs. ≤1	4,2	1,14-15,50	**0,031**	1,5	0,40-5,58	0,547	4,3	1,25-15,0	**0,021**	4,0	1,20-13,49	**0,024**
R^2	$R^2 = 0,44$			$R^2 = 0,19$			$R^2 = 0,39$			$R^2 = 0,45$		

1 adjustiert für Alter, Schmerzen T_0, körperliche Belastung, Intervention
2 adjustiert für Alter, Schmerzen T_0, körperliche Belastung, Intervention, OVC, Handlungsspielraum
3 adjustiert für Alter, Schmerzen T_0, körperliche Belastung, Intervention
4 adjustiert für Alter, Schmerzen T_0, körperliche Belastung, Intervention, Handlungsspielraum, Sport, Konflikte mit Eltern

Die logtransformierte ERI-Variable hatte einen erhöhenden, statistisch signifikanten Einfluss auf das Burnout. Übertragen auf das entlogarithmierte Skalenniveau würde sich bei einer Erhöhung des ERI-Quotienten um 10 % der Burnout-Wert um 1,1 Punkte erhöhen (95 %-CI: 0,09-2,14, p = 0,034) (Tabelle 5). Weiterhin konnte beobachtet werden, dass für Beschäftigte aus Kitas im Vergleich zu Beschäftigten aus den beiden anderen Einrichtungsarten der Burnout-Wert im Mittel um 7 Punkte höher war (95 %-CI: 0,56-13,51). Diese Erhöhung war statistisch signifikant (p = 0,034). Eine Interaktion von ERI und OVC war auch in diesem Fall nicht zu beobachten.

Tabelle 5 Ergebnisse der multivariaten linearen Regression für Burnout (adjustiert für Burnout T_0, Teilnahme an Otoplastikenstudie)

R^2:0,53		Regressions-koeffizient	Standardisierter Beta-Koeffizient	95%-CI	p
Erhöhung des ERI-Quotienten um 10%		1,1	0,18	0,09-2,14	**0,034**
Kindertagesstätte vs. andere Einrichtungen		7,0	0,16	0,56-13,51	**0,034**
Vielseitigkeit (Skala 1-5)		-3,8	-0,14	-8,0-0,37	0,074
Alter (pro Jahr)		0,6	-,029	0,87- -0,29	**0,001**

1.4.4 Diskussion

Muskuloskelettale Beschwerden

Im Längsschnitt wurden bei Erzieher/-innen statistisch signifikante Assoziationen zwischen einem erhöhten ERI-Quotienten und der Zunahme von MSB in drei von vier Körperregionen festgestellt: Kreuz, Nacken und die Kombination von mindestens einer der drei Körperregionen (MSB gesamt). Dabei wurde für den Confounder körperliche Belastungen kontrolliert.

Der hier im Längsschnitt beobachtete Zusammenhang von ERI und Kreuzschmerzen bei Erzieher/-innen (OR: 4,2) wurde ebenfalls in Längsschnittstudien bei Beschäftigten aus anderen Branchen (Fahrer eines Verkehrsunternehmens, Beschäftigte in der öffentlichen Verwaltung) beobachtet (Rugulies 2008; Lapointe 2013). In Querschnittsstudien ist dieser Zusammenhang bei Beschäftigten aus der Pflege, dem Weinanbau, der Polizei und einem öffentlichen Verkehrsunternehmen beobachtet worden (Dragano 2003; von dem Knesebeck 2005; Simon 2008; Bernard 2011). In Bezug auf Nackenschmerzen zeigte sich ERI ebenfalls als ein statistisch signifikanter Prädiktor (OR: 4,3). Dieser Effekt wurde auch bei Fahrern und Bürobeschäftigten im Längsschnitt (Rugulies 2008; Lapointe 2013) sowie bei Beschäftigten aus Krankenhäusern bzw. dem Weinanbau im Querschnitt beobachtet (Gillen 2007; Simon 2008; Bernard 2011).

Auch bei der Kombinationsvariable MSB gesamt war ERI ein statistisch signifikanter Einflussfaktor (OR: 4,0). Es zeigte sich auch, dass zwei weitere Variablen, Konflikte mit Eltern (OR: 4,9) sowie sportliche Aktivität (OR: 0,3), einen statistisch signifikanten Einfluss auf MSB gesamt hatten. Hinweise einer Interaktion von ERI und OVC ließen sich bei keiner der Körperregionen feststellen; bislang wurde nur eine Querschnittsuntersuchung publiziert, die einen solchen Interaktionseffekt bei Krankenschwestern fand (Weyers 2006).

Aus Sicht betrieblicher Prävention liefern die Ergebnisse den Hinweis, dass anhand des ERI-Fragebogens frühzeitig Beschäftigte identifiziert werden könnten, die ein erhöhtes MSB-Risiko haben. Weiterhin sprechen die Ergebnisse für die Durchführung von Seminaren zum Konfliktmanagement. Dadurch würden Erzieher/-innen nicht nur fachlich weitergebildet, sondern sie würden auch lernen, Belastungen in Konfliktsituationen besser zu vermeiden. Möglicherweise könnte auf diesem Weg die Entstehung oder Chronifizierung von MSB ebenfalls verhindert werden. Auch legen die Ergebnisse nahe, dass z. B. betriebssportliche Angebote sich positiv auf den Muskel- und Skelettapparat auswirken. Solche Angebote könnten auch als Belohnung wahrgenommen werden und das Wertschätzungsempfinden der Beschäftigten fördern und somit das Entstehen beruflicher Gratifikationskrisen vermeiden. Auf diese Weise könnten sich betriebssportliche Angebote möglicherweise in zweifacher Hinsicht auf die Entstehung von MSB positiv auswirken.

Burnout

Die Ergebnisse der linearen Regression zeigten, dass eine Erhöhung des ERI-Quotienten eine statistisch signifikante Erhöhung des Burnout-Werts zur Folge hat (bei einer relativen Erhöhung des ERI-Quotienten um 10 % stieg der Burnout-Wert um 1,1 Punkte).

Dieses Ergebnis deckt sich mit einer Längsschnittuntersuchung bei Pflegedienstleitungen (Spence 2008) sowie weiteren Querschnittsstudien bei Erzieher/-innen und Lehrer/-innen (Scheuch 2007; Loerbroks 2014; Gluschkoff 2016). Auch bei Krankenhausärzten finden Klein et al. den erhöhenden Einfluss von ERI auf Burnout (Klein 2010). Nach Siegrist gilt das Persönlichkeitsmerkmal OVC als ein guter Prädiktor für Burnout, der in einer Reihe von Studien bestätigt wird (Lau 2008; Nübling 2013; Chou 2014; Wang 2015). Entgegen dieser Beobachtungen gab es in der vorliegenden Arbeit keinen Zusammenhang zwischen OVC und Burnout. Weiterhin ergab die Analyse, dass Erzieher/-innen aus Kitas einen durchschnittlich um 7 Punkte höheren Burnout-Wert hatten als die Beschäftigten aus den Schulkooperationen und Jugendeinrichtungen. Die aus der Gefährdungsbeurteilung resultierenden Maßnahmen zur Burnout-Prävention sollten demnach insbesondere bei den Kita-Erzieher/-innen durchgeführt werden. Dies bestätigt einen Teil der Schlussfolgerungen aus Studie 1.

1.5 Studie 3 – Use of Moulded Hearing Protectors by Child Care Workers - An Interventional Pilot Study (Otoplastikenstudie)

1.5.1 Studienziel

Maßnahmen zur Lärmprävention in Kitas finden auf technisch-organisatorischer Ebene statt. Sie beinhalten z. B. die Auswahl von speziellem Spielzeug und Mobiliar, den Ausbau von Lärmdämmungen, den Einsatz von Lärmampeln, die Einrichtung von Rückzugsräumen für das Personal oder die Lärmerziehung der Kinder. In der Industrie werden neben technisch-organisatorischen auch persönliche Maßnahmen zur Prävention von Gehörschäden ergriffen. Ein individueller Gehörschutz ist bei einem mittleren Tages-Lärmexpositionspegel von über 80 dB(A) in Deutschland auf Basis der EG-Lärmrichtlinie 2003/10/EG durch die Lärm- und Vibrations-Arbeitsschutzverordnung durch den Arbeitgeber bereitzustellen, sofern technisch-organisatorische Maßnahmen die Lärmemission nicht weiter verringern können (EU 2003; LärmVibrationsArbSchV 2007). Beschäftigte z. B. beim Militär, in der Landwirtschaft oder in der Industrie tragen häufig einen Kapselgehörschutz zur Vorbeugung von Lärmschwerhörigkeit (Erlandsson 1980; Brink 2002; Berg 2009; Heyer 2011; Verbeek 2014). Berufsmusiker benutzen häufig Otoplastiken, die aufgrund von regelbaren Filtersystemen im Vergleich zum Kapselgehörschutz den Vorteil haben, dass die Sprachverständlichkeit erhalten bleibt. Otoplastiken werden teilweise auch bei einer Überempfindlichkeit gegenüber Lärm (Hyperakusis) selektiv bei Lehrer/-innen und Erzieher/-innen eingesetzt.

Den Beschäftigten des Trägers für Kinder- und Jugendeinrichtungen wurde eine betriebliche Lärmpräventionsmaßnahme in Form einer Pilotstudie angeboten, die anhand folgender Studienfragen evaluiert wurde:

1a) Reduziert der Einsatz von Otoplastiken die subjektive Lärmbelastung bei Erzieher/-innen?

1b) Reduziert der Einsatz von Otoplastiken das Burnout-Risiko bei Erzieher/-innen?

2) Wie sind die akustischen Gegebenheiten in kritischen Räumen? Gibt es Assoziationen zwischen den akustischen Gegebenheiten der Räume und subjektiver Lärmbelastung bzw. Burnout?

3) Halten Erzieher/-innen den Einsatz von Otoplastiken für geeignet?

1.5.2 Methoden

Im Rahmen einer Interventionsstudie mit Vorher-Nachher-Vergleich (Follow-up: zwölf Monate) wurde allen pädagogischen MitarbeiterInnen des Trägers (N = 400) die Teilnahme an der Studie angeboten (Abbildung 7); 45 Beschäftigte aus 16 verschiedenen Einrichtungen willigten ein. Um die Ergebnisse aus einer weiteren Perspektive interpretieren zu können, wurde post-hoc eine Vergleichsgruppe aus denjenigen gebildet, die keine Otoplastiken trugen und nur an der Kohortenstudie (Studie 2) teilnahmen. Diese zusätzliche Betrachtung wurde gewählt, um beurteilen zu können, ob das Belastungspotenzial für diejenigen ohne Intervention konstant geblieben ist oder sich über die Zeit verändert hat. Da es sich bei dieser Gruppe nicht um eine klassische Kontrollgruppe handelte, wird im Folgenden der Begriff Referenzgruppe verwendet. Beschäftigte aus Einrichtungen der Kinder- und Jugendförderung (Wohngruppen, Jugendprojekte) wurden aus diesem Vergleich ausgeschlossen (N = 12), da in der Interventionsgruppe keiner aus diesen Einrichtungen stammte.

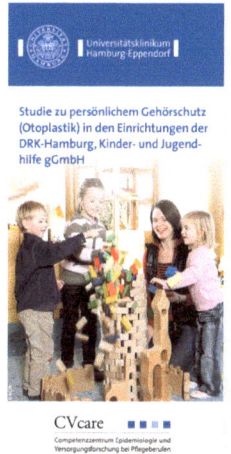

Die Teilnehmer/innen erhielten persönlich angepasste Otoplastiken (Variphone „MEP-2G" Hearing Protector) und nahmen zu Beginn der Studie an einem Workshop zum Umgang mit Otoplastiken und Lärm teil. Über die gesamte Beobachtungszeit dokumentierten sie ihre Tragezeiten in einem Tagebuch. Zusätzlich zu dem in Kapitel 1.3.2 beschriebenen Fragebogen erhielten sie einen Fragebogen

Abbildung 7 Flyer zur Otoplastikenstudie

zur Nutzungszufriedenheit. Dieser erhob fünf Monate (T$_0$ + fünf Monate) und zwölf Monate nach Interventionsbeginn (T1) Informationen zu dem Tragekomfort, der akustischen Wahrnehmung und der Sinnhaftigkeit des Tragens der Otoplastiken während der Arbeit. Die Antworten sind auf Basis einer fünfstufigen Ratingskala erhoben und im Anschluss dichotomisiert worden.

Um neben der subjektiven Lärmbelastung auch objektive Daten zu der Raumakustik zu gewinnen, wurden während des Beobachtungszeitraums in kritischen Räumen Nachhallzeiten gemessen. Die Messungen in Räumen mit unterschiedlicher Funktionalität (Spiel- und Gruppenräume, Klassenzimmer, Bewegungsräume, Treppenhäuser, Kinderrestaurants) erfolgten im Frequenzbereich von 125 bis 4000 Hertz. Die Ergebnisse wurden mit den Sollwerten der „DIN-Norm 18041 – Hörsamkeit in kleinen bis mittelgroßen Räumen" verglichen (DIN 2015). Ein Raumakustiker beurteilte abschließend auf Basis der Nachhallzeiten und der baulichen Eigenschaften die entsprechenden Räume. Es wurden zwischen ein und vier Räume pro Einrichtung begutachtet, für eine Einrichtung konnte aus organisatorischen Gründen keine Begutachtung durchgeführt werden.

1.5.3 Ergebnisse

Nach der Follow-up-Zeit von zwölf Monaten waren von den anfänglich 45 Proband/-innen insgesamt 33 Fragebögen eingegangen (Follow-up-Rate: 73 %). Zum Zeitpunkt der Baseline waren 91 % Frauen (n = 41) unter den Proband/-innen, die Altersgruppe der 40- bis 50-Jährigen war mit 38 % am stärksten vertreten (n = 17). In Vollzeit arbeiteten zu diesem Zeitpunkt 40 % (n = 18), 80 % der Gruppe waren in Kitas beschäftigt (n = 36).

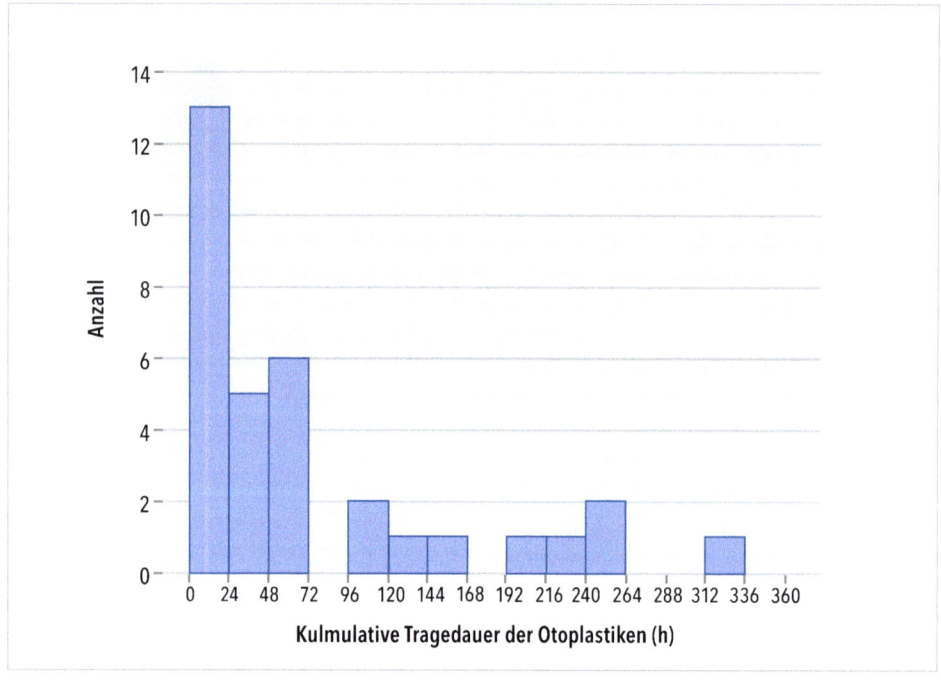

Abbildung 8 Über zwölf Monate kumulierte Tragezeit der Otoplastiken (N = 33)

Der Median der kumulierten Tragezeit in Stunden betrug 34,6 (Range: 0–326) (Abbildung 8). Die Anzahl der kumulierten Tage, an denen die Otoplastiken eingesetzt wurden, lag im Median bei 32 (Range: 0–174 Tage). Auf Individualbasis wurde jedoch beobachtet, dass die persönlichen täglichen Tragezeiten über den Beobachtungszeitraum immer weiter abnahmen.

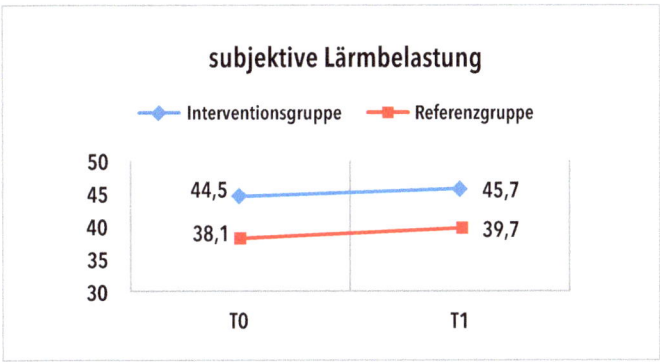

Abbildung 9 Entwicklung der subjektiven Lärmbelastung in Intervention- und Referenzgruppe (Wertebereich: 13-65)

Der Vergleich von Interventions- und Referenzgruppe zum Zeitpunkt T_0 zeigte bezüglich der demografischen Variablen und aller Einflussvariablen keine statistisch signifikanten Unterschiede. Der einzige statistisch signifikante Unterschied zwischen den Gruppen wurde in Bezug auf subjektive Lärmbelastung beobachtet ($p = 0,004$). Die subjektive Lärmbelastung in der Interventionsgruppe wies einen mittleren Anstieg von 44,5 auf 45,7 Punkte auf (Abbildung 9). Die Differenz in der subjektiven Lärmbelastung war in der Referenzgruppe höher (ΔT_1-T_0 = 1,6 vs. 1,2) als in der Interventionsgruppe. Der Unterschied der Differenzen zwischen den Gruppen war statistisch nicht signifikant ($p = 0,8$).

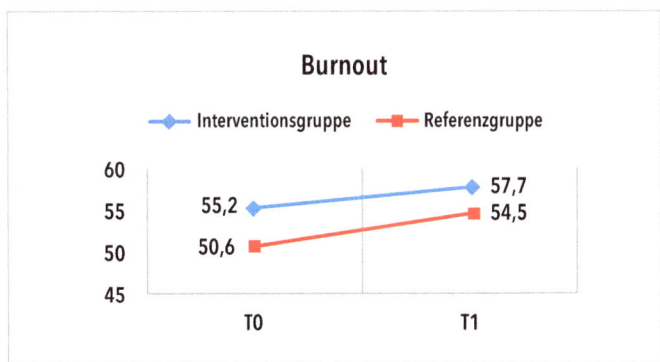

Abbildung 10 Entwicklung von Burnout in Intervention- und Referenzgruppe (Wertebereich: 0-100)

Hinsichtlich des Burnout-Risikos zeigte sich bei der Interventionsgruppe ein Anstieg von 55,2 auf 57,7 Punkte ($\Delta = 2,5$) (Abbildung 10). Der Anstieg in der Referenzgruppe von 50,6 auf 54,5 Punkte war größer ($\Delta = 3,9$) und statistisch signifikant ($p = 0,05$). Der Unterschied zwischen den Differenzen zwischen den Gruppen war statistisch nicht signifikant ($p = 0,7$).

Verteilt auf 15 Einrichtungen (elf Kitas, vier Schulkooperationen) wurden insgesamt in 39 kritischen Räumen Nachhallzeitmessungen durchgeführt. In 29 Räumen (74 %) lagen die Nachhallzeiten über den individuellen Sollwerten, die nach DIN-Norm abhängig von Funktionalität und Größe der Räume sind (DIN 2015). Unter Berücksichtigung dieser Messungen und weiterer akustischer Merkmale empfahl der Raumakustiker für neun von 15 Einrichtungen für mindestens einen Raum akustische Verbesserungsmaßnahmen.

Zum Zeitpunkt des Follow-up zeigte sich, dass die Burnout-Werte von Proband/-innen in Einrichtungen mit einer schlechten raumakustischen Beurteilung höher lagen (Abbildung 11a und b) als bei den Personen aus Einrichtungen mit guter Raumakustik ($\bar{x}$: 60,8 vs. 52,1). Dieselbe Tendenz gab es auch bei der subjektiven Lärmbelastung. Hier wiesen diejenigen aus Einrichtungen mit guter Akustik einen geringeren Mittelwert auf ($\bar{x}$: 42,8) als diejenigen aus Einrichtungen mit schlechter Akustik ($\bar{x}$: 47,7). Die Unterschiede bei beiden Variablen waren statistisch nicht signifikant.

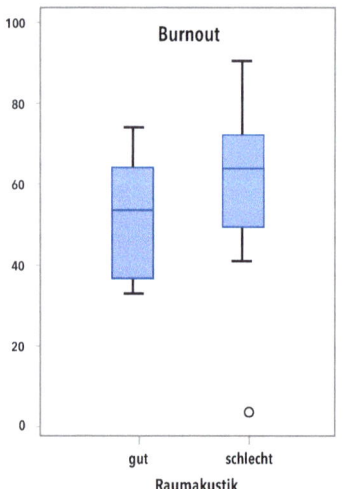 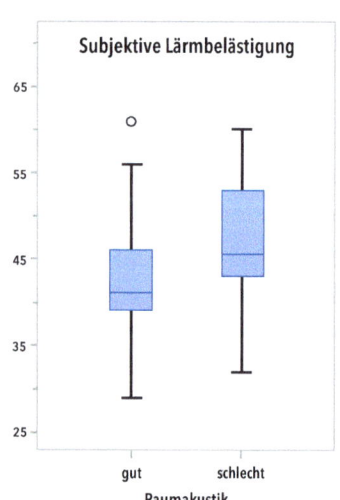

Abbildung 11a und 11b Burnout bzw. subjektive Lärmbelastung nach Einrichtung mit raumakustischer Beurteilung zum Zeitpunkt T1

Die Zufriedenheit mit den Otoplastiken nahm im Zeitverlauf tendenziell ab (Abbildung 12). Der Anteil derjenigen, denen das Tragen des Gehörschutzes in Anwesenheit von Eltern unangenehm war, erhöhte sich von 18 % auf 35 %. Der Anteil derjenigen, die das Tragen von Otoplastiken als sinnvoll empfanden, sank von 69 % auf 47 %. Der Anteil derjenigen, die sich nach der Arbeit entspannter fühlten, blieb konstant (48 %). Der Anteil der Proband/-innen, der angab, dass Informationen entgehen würden, reduzierte sich von 27 % auf 23 %. Nach fünf Monaten gaben rund drei Viertel (72 %) der Proband/-innen an, weiterhin ihren pädagogischen Auftrag erfüllen zu können, zum Zeitpunkt T1 waren es noch 67 %. Alle Verläufe waren statistisch nicht signifikant.

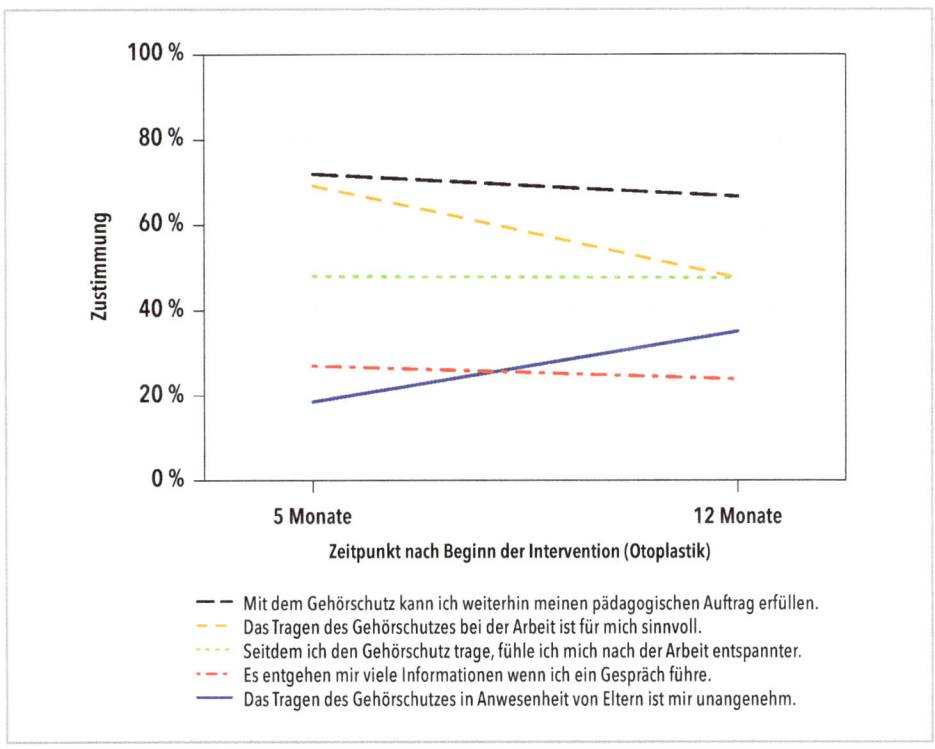

Abbildung 12 Zufriedenheit mit den Otoplastiken fünf und zwölf Monate nach Interventionsbeginn

1.5.4 Diskussion

Der Einsatz von Otoplastiken bei Erzieher/-innen konnte die subjektive Lärm-belastung und das Burnout-Risiko nicht nachweisbar reduzieren. Weiterhin wurde eine Abnahme der Zufriedenheit mit dem Tragen von Otoplastiken beobachtet. Bei mehr als der Hälfte der Einrichtungen wurden akustische Verbesserungen empfoh-len. In den betroffenen Einrichtungen waren Burnout und subjektive Lärmbelastung bei den Proband/-innen tendenziell höher ausgeprägt.

Ausgehend von dem Medianwert der kumulierten Tragezeit (34 Stunden in zwölf Monaten) ergab sich bei Annahme einer Vollbeschäftigung (224 Arbeitstage im Jahr 2015) eine mittlere tägliche Tragezeit von maximal neun Minuten für die Hälfte der Proband/-innen. Da keine Studien zu dem Effekt von Otoplastiken publiziert waren, war es schwierig, ohne Referenzwerte zu beurteilen, ob es sich dabei um eine in Bezug auf Lärmprävention effektive Zeitspanne handelte. In dem anfänglichen Workshop wurde den Proband/-innen zwar geraten, die Otoplastiken insbesondere zu den Lärmspitzenzeiten zu tragen. Vor dem Hintergrund der zunehmenden Un-zufriedenheit mit den Otoplastiken (pädagogischer Auftrag, Sinnhaftigkeit, Ent-spannungseffekt) haben die Proband/-innen die Geräte möglicherweise bewusst wenig getragen, weil diese bei der Arbeit störten. Dafür sprachen auch die abneh-menden individuellen Tragezeiten. Qualitative Forschung in Form von persönlichen Interviews hätte die Gründe für die geringen Tragezeiten deutlicher herausarbeiten können.

Die raumakustische Begutachtung stellte bei neun von 15 Einrichtungen Ver-besserungspotenzial fest. Im Einzelnen ging es um raumakustische Gegebenheiten, die trotz teilweise moderater Nachhallzeiten als verbesserungswürdig angesehen wurden. Dabei handelte es sich z. B. um fehlende oder falsch montierte Schall-absorberelemente, fehlende Trittschalldämmung, zu viele glatte Oberflächen, feh-lende Rückzugsbereiche oder laut schließende Metalltüren. Ein weiterer Kritikpunkt des Raumakustikers war die Beobachtung, dass sich teilweise zu viele Kinder auf zu engem Raum befanden; seiner Einschätzung nach würden sich in dieser Situa-tion akustische Verbesserungsmaßnahmen ab einem gewissen Punkt als erfolglos erweisen.

Die subjektiv erhobenen Outcomes wurden durch die tendenziellen Unter-schiede zwischen Beschäftigten aus den Einrichtungen mit bzw. ohne raumakustischem Verbesserungspotenzial bestätigt. Dies spricht tendenziell gegen eine Antwortverzerrung aufgrund sozialer Erwünschtheit. Gezielte Verbesserungsmaßnahmen in den betroffenen Einrichtungen würden somit den am stärksten belasteten Personen zugutekommen. Studien zeigen, dass aufgrund raumakustischer Verbesserungen die Nachhallzeiten und teilweise auch die subjektive Lärmbelastung in pädagogischen Einrichtungen gesenkt werden konnten (Truchnon-Gagnon 1988; Gerhardsson 2013; Sjodin 2014). Auch der Einsatz von speziellen Spielzeugbehältern senkte den Schalldruckpegel erheblich (Scharf 2015). Zudem gibt es über die baulichen Maßnahmen hinaus auf organisatorischer Ebene Möglichkeiten, die Lärmbelastung zu reduzieren. Dazu gehören beispielsweise das Nutzen von Erholungsräumen, der Einsatz einer Lärmampel, eine Lichtregulierung, eine lärmsensibilisierende Pädagogik sowie ein spezielles Sprechtraining für Erzieher/-innen.

Die Ergebnisse dieser Studie verdeutlichen, dass das Tragen von Otoplastiken in diesem speziellen Setting keine effektive und arbeitsgerechte Maßnahme war und aus diesem Grunde möglicherweise auch nicht gut implementiert werden konnte. Es zeigte sich auch, dass die vorliegenden technisch-organisatorischen Verhältnisse in Bezug auf Lärmprävention nicht optimal ausgestaltet waren.

1.6 Diskussion

Die drei vorgestellten Studien geben Einblick in das Belastungs- und Bean-spruchungsempfinden sowie in die Durchführung einer betrieblichen Intervention zu Lärm von Erzieher/-innen. In der ersten Studie wurde eine im Vergleich zu aktuellen Studien ähnlich hohe ERI-Prävalenz bei Erzieher/-innen beobachtet (Viernickel 2013; Schreyer 2014). Im Vergleich zu anderen Studien gab es eine überdurchschnittlich hohe Prävalenz von Burnout (Buch 2001; Rudow 2004; Jungbauer 2015). Für die Subgruppe der Beschäftigten aus den Kitas wurden in Bezug auf ERI und Burnout die höchsten Ausprägungen festgestellt.

In der zweiten Studie ließ sich im Längsschnitt ein statistisch signifikanter Effekt von ERI auf die Zunahme von MSB nachweisen. Dies gilt für Kreuz- und Nacken-schmerzen sowie für die Kombination von Kreuz-, Schulter- oder Nackenschmerzen. Ebenfalls gab es in der Studie einen statistisch signifikanten Zusammenhang zwischen ERI und Burnout bei Erzieher/-innen.

In der Studie 3 wurde deutlich, dass subjektive Lärmbelastung sowie Burnout durch das Tragen von Otoplastiken nicht statistisch nachweisbar reduziert werden konnte. Zudem kam es zu einer abnehmenden Zufriedenheit mit dem Einsatz von Otoplastiken. Ebenfalls wurde festgestellt, dass bei 60% der Einrichtungen raum-akustische Defizite vorlagen und dass dort die subjektive Lärmbelastung und das Burnout der Studienteilnehmer/-innen tendenziell höher ausfielen.

Bei den Beschäftigten wurde in der vorliegenden Arbeit eine hohe Prävalenz von ERI beobachtet, die über die Beobachtungszeit weiter angestiegen ist (Baseline: 65%, $\bar{x}$: 1,2, Follow-up: 87%; $\bar{x}$: 1,3). Unter Einbezug früherer Studien bei deutschen Erzieher/-innen ist längerfristig eine tendenzielle Erhöhung der ERI-Prävalenzen bzw. der Mittelwerte festzustellen (Tabelle 6). Die subjektiv wahrgenommene psychosoziale Belastung der Erzieher/-innen in Deutschland hat sich somit in dem Erhebungszeitraum 2003 bis 2015 deutlich erhöht.

Tabelle 6 Publikationen mit ERI-Schätzungen bei Erzieher/-innen in dem Zeitraum 2003–2015

Erhebungs-zeitpunkt	2003 (Scheuch 2007)	2007 (Nübling 2013)	2010 (Viernickel 2013)	2012 (Schreyer 2014)	2014 (Koch 2015)	2015 (Koch 2017)
N	150	nicht berichtet	1958	6518	199	106
ERI-Prävalenz	-	-	64%	67%	65%	87%
ERI-Quotient Mittelwert	0,5	0,6	1,3	1,3	1,17	1,3

Wie eingangs bereits erwähnt, haben sich parallel zu diesem Zeitraum die strukturellen Rahmenbedingungen im Kita-Bereich verändert. Nach der Verabschiedung des „Gemeinsamen Rahmens der Länder für die frühe Bildung in Kindertageseinrichtungen" im Jahre 2004 sollten Erzieher/innen neue Aufgaben übernehmen., z. B. die naturwissenschaftliche, mathematische und technische Bildung, die Sprachförderung und das Beobachten und Dokumentieren des Entwicklungsstands der einzelnen Kinder (Jugendministerkonferenz 2004). Hieraus resultierte für Erzieher/-innen ein großer Qualifikationsbedarf, der neben der pädagogischen Arbeit erfüllt werden sollte. Eine aktuelle Untersuchung zeigt, dass Erzieher/-innen immer noch vor einem Umsetzungsdilemma stehen, da nach wie vor eine Diskrepanz zwischen den pädagogischen Forderungen der Bildungsprogramme der Bundesländer und den Arbeitsbedingungen herrscht (Viernickel 2013).

Zum Zweiten wurde im Jahr 2013 ein Gesetz wirksam, das, neben dem damals schon bestehenden rechtlichen Anspruch auf Betreuung für Kinder im Alter von drei bis sechs Jahren, den Betreuungsanspruch für Kinder von ein bis unter drei Jahren regelt (SGB VIII 2008). Der Anteil der betreuten Kinder in diesem Alter ist von 2006 bis 2016 von 9 % auf 18 % gestiegen (Statistisches Bundesamt 2016). Die daraus resultierende Arbeitslast ist nicht äquivalent mit dem gleichen Anstieg von Kindern im Alter von drei bis sechs Jahren: im Bundesdurchschnitt liegt für Krippenkinder ein Erzieher/-innen-Kind-Schlüssel von 1:4,3 vor, für Kinder im Alter von drei bis sechs Jahren liegt dieser bei 1:9,2 (Bock-Famulla 2017). Resultierend aus diesen veränderten strukturellen Rahmenbedingungen kam es für das pädagogische Kita-Personal in den vergangenen zehn Jahren zu einer deutlich zunehmenden Arbeitsbelastung, die nicht durch wesentliche Gratifikationen ausgeglichen wurde. In den aktuellsten Umfragen bewerten 71% der Erzieher/-innen ihr Gehalt als zu niedrig und ca. die Hälfte der befragten Träger einer Studie geben an, überwiegend befristet einzustellen (Viernickel 2013; Schreyer 2014).

Die in Studie 1 beobachteten Belastungen durch Lärm, zu große Gruppengrößen und ERI sollten vor dem Hintergrund dieser veränderten Rahmenbedingungen betrachtet werden. Dennoch kann in dieser Arbeit kein empirischer Bezug zwischen veränderten strukturellen Rahmenbedingungen und den etwaigen daraus resultierenden Belastungen hergestellt werden. Es gibt empirische Hinweise, dass ungünstige Rahmenbedingungen in Kitas, die zwischen Kommunen oder Ländern variieren können, mit einer erhöhten ERI-Prävalenz assoziiert sind. Viernickel et al. beobachteten, dass ein ungünstiger struktureller Rahmenbedingungsindex in Kitas (Index bestehend aus: Erzieher/-innen-Kind-Schlüssel, Gruppengröße, Ausmaß der Fluktuation, Aspekte der Raumgestaltung, Umfang an mittelbarer Arbeit, Einkommen) nicht nur mit ERI korreliert ist, sondern auch mit Burnout, MSB, psychischen Beeinträchtigungen und der Arbeitsfähigkeit (Viernickel 2013).

Der im Längsschnitt beobachtete Zusammenhang von ERI und MSB bei Erzieher/-innen ergänzt den geringen und kontroversen Forschungsstand zu diesem Thema. Allerdings muss diese epidemiologische Erkenntnis mit Vorsicht gedeutet werden, da MSB auch in Verbindung mit einer Reihe anderer Faktoren stehen kann, die hier nicht berücksichtigt wurden, wie z.B. biomechanische oder psychosoziale Belastungen im Privatleben oder eine genetische Prädisposition. Angesichts des Zusammenhangs von ERI mit MSB und Burnout wird deutlich, welches Potenzial die Prävention dieser psychosozialen Belastungen darstellt. Die in Studie 1 und anderen Untersuchungen beobachteten gut ausgebildeten Ressourcen bei Erzieher/-innen sind eine gute Voraussetzung für die Durchführung betrieblicher Interventionen (Berger 2002; Rudow 2005; Fuchs 2008). Mit Blick auf den stresstheoretischen Erklärungsansatz des ERI-Modells stellen die Skalen Anforderung und Belohnung bzw. die Belohnungssubskalen Gehalt, Wertschätzung/Anerkennung und Arbeitsplatzsicherheit/Aufstiegsmöglichkeiten Ansatzpunkte für präventive Maßnahmen dar. Die ERI-Prävention durch modellbasierte betriebliche Interventionsmaßnahmen wurde in internationalen Studien untersucht (Aust 1997; Bourbonnais 2006; Limm 2011; Bourbonnais 2011). Diese Programme erwiesen sich als geeignet, da sie die psychosoziale Arbeitsumgebung und die mentale Gesundheit positiv beeinflussten. So beeinflussten Interventionen auf der individuellen und organisatorischen Ebene das OVC bei Busfahrern positiv (Aust 1997), reduzierten die negativen psychologischen Anforderungen bei Beschäftigten in

Krankenhäusern langfristig (Bourbonnais 2011) und senkten die Stressreaktivität bei Beschäftigten im unteren Management signifikant (Limm 2011). Dennoch ist der Forschungsstand bei diesen Interventionen zu gering, um eine verlässliche Aussage zur Evidenz zu machen. Veränderungen der Belohnungskomponenten Gehalt und Arbeitsplatzsicherheit/Aufstiegsmöglichkeiten sind auf betrieblicher Ebene für Erzieher/-innen kaum durchführbar, da die Finanzierung des Kita-Personals hauptsächlich durch die Kommunen und Länder erfolgt. Hinsichtlich der fehlenden Wertschätzung aber, die in Studie 2 deutlich wurde, gibt es auf betrieblicher Ebene die Möglichkeit, Teams und insbesondere Führungskräfte durch Seminare für Wertschätzungsfragen zu sensibilisieren. In einer Beobachtungsstudie wurde festgestellt, dass Beschäftigte, die in Betrieben mit einer guten Wertschätzungskultur arbeiten, gesünder und leistungsfähiger sind (Hinding 2012). Bei Büroangestellten z. B. konnte durch eine Intervention die wahrgenommene Wertschätzung erhöht und die Prävalenz von MSB gesenkt werden (Gilbert-Ouimet 2011).

Die Schwierigkeit, die Lärmbelastung von Erzieher/-innen durch verhaltenspräventive Maßnahmen zu senken, wurde in Studie 3 deutlich. Es konnte keine Reduzierung in den Zielvariablen festgestellt werden, die Zufriedenheit mit den Otoplastiken nahm über die Zeit ab. Parallel wurde durch die raumakustische Begutachtung deutlich, dass mögliche Maßnahmen zur Lärmprävention auf der technisch-organisatorischen Ebene nicht voll ausgeschöpft bzw. falsch durchgeführt wurden. Der interventionelle Teil der Studie war somit ein Versuch, die Lärmbelastung der Beschäftigten symptomatisch zu behandeln. Dies widerspricht dem § 4 des im Arbeitsschutzgesetz verankerten Grundsatzes, Gefährdungen nach Möglichkeit an der Quelle zu bekämpfen und individuelle Schutzmaßnahmen als nachrangig zu betrachten (ArbSchG 1996). Dort wird die Rangfolge der Maßnahmen dem TOP-Prinzip folgend erläutert: Vorrang haben technische Maßnahmen (T), sind diese nicht ausreichend, werden sie durch organisatorische ergänzt (O) und als letzte zusätzliche Option erfolgen personenbezogenen Maßnahmen (P). Diese aufbauende Abfolge von Lärmpräventionsmaßnahmen lag offensichtlich nur bei einem Teil der Einrichtungen vor, sodass es bei der Mehrheit ein raumakustisches Verbesserungspotenzial gab. Die Ergebnisse verdeutlichen, dass bei einem Träger für Kinder- und Jugendeinrichtungen ein professionelles Raumakustikkonzept die Lärmbelastung des Personals reduzieren könnte. Dennoch sollten diese Ergebnisse ebenfalls vor dem Hintergrund der Veränderung der strukturellen Rahmenbedingungen von Kitas betrachtet werden.

Limitationen

Eine Limitation der Arbeit waren die geringen Fallzahlen. Hieraus ergaben sich weite Konfidenzintervalle und ungenaue Schätzungen der Punktschätzer. Weiterhin sind die Odds Ratios aus der Kohortenstudie wegen der hohen MSB-Prävalenzraten überschätzt und sollten daher mit Vorsicht interpretiert werden. Aufgrund des Auswahlverfahrens ist die Stichprobe der Erzieher/-innen nicht repräsentativ für Hamburg. Im Vergleich zu einer repräsentativen Studie über deutsche Erzieher/-innen ließen sich aber keine Unterschiede bezüglich des Alters, Geschlechts und der Nationalität nachweisen (Schreyer, Krause et al. 2014). Einfluss- und Outcome-Variablen entstammten aus derselben Quelle – eine Verzerrung durch Einheitsmethodenvarianz kann hier, z. B. durch soziale Erwünschtheit, nicht ausgeschlossen werden (Podsakoff 2003). Im Verlauf zeigten sich in Studie 1 bzw. 2 hohe und ansteigende Prävalenzraten von Burnout und ERI. Aufgrund einer nicht vorhersehbaren Streikwelle zu den Erhebungszeitpunkten 2014 und 2015 kann ein Klassifikationsbias von ERI und auch Burnout nicht ausgeschlossen werden. Es ist durchaus vorstellbar, dass die berufspolitische Situation der Erzieher/-innen in Deutschland die StudienteilnehmerInnen in ihrem Antwortverhalten sensibilisiert hat. Anders als bei einem klassischen RCT wurde die Interventionsstudie ohne Kontrollgruppe, ohne Randomisierung und ohne Monitoring der sonstigen Bedingungen durchgeführt. Die Post-hoc-Analyse, das Einbeziehen und der Vergleich mit der Referenzgruppe veranschaulichte, in welchem Ausmaß die Studie unter sich ändernden, nicht kontrollierten Bedingungen stattfand. Die betriebliche Präventionsmaßnahme gegen Lärm, die aus ethischen Gründen allen Beschäftigten zugänglich sein sollte, stand in Konkurrenz zu den Kriterien einer wissenschaftlichen Untersuchung. Fehlende spezifische Ein- und Ausschlusskriterien (z. B. Hörstatus) führten zur einer Selbstselektion der Proband/-innen. Eine Heterogenität des Studienkollektivs kann demnach nicht ausgeschlossen werden. Weiterhin hätte ein qualitativer Forschungsstrang die Gründe für die geringe Compliance sowie für die Unzufriedenheit mit dem Tragen von Otoplastiken deutlicher herausarbeiten können.

1.7 Fazit

Das Ziel der vorliegenden Arbeit war es, bestimmte gesundheitliche Belastungen von Erzieher/-innen (MSB und Burnout) zu erheben und in Relation zu ERI zu setzen. Weiterhin sollte die Präventionsmöglichkeit von Burnout und subjektiver Lärmbelastung durch das Tragen von Otoplastiken untersucht werden.

Unter Berücksichtigung der Limitationen werden in dieser Arbeit Erzieher/-innen als eine psychosozial stark belastete Berufsgruppe identifiziert, die durch ein ungünstiges Verhältnis von Anforderungen und Belohnungen gekennzeichnet ist. Im Vergleich zu Studienergebnissen aus den vergangenen zehn Jahren hat sich der Anteil psychosozial belasteter Erzieher/-innen erhöht. Der quantitative und der qualitative Ausbau von Kitas sollten von strukturellen Änderungen begleitet werden, die zu mehr Personal, zu einer Reduktion der Gruppengrößen und zu einer höheren monetären und nicht monetären Wertschätzung und zu gesellschaftlicher Anerkennung führen.

Der beobachtete Zusammenhang von ERI und MSB bzw. Burnout gibt Hinweise auf mögliche Folgen der psychosozialen Belastung durch ERI. Auf dieser Grundlage könnte der ERI-Fragebogen als potenzielles arbeitsmedizinisches Screening-Instrument für Erzieher/-innen, die ein erhöhtes gesundheitliches Risiko haben, eingesetzt werden. Eine weitergehende wissenschaftliche Untersuchung zu diesem Thema ist aber wichtig, um eine belastbare Aussage zu der Evidenz machen zu können.

Der Versuch, die Lärmbelastung von Erzieher/-innen durch persönlichen Gehörschutz zu reduzieren, stieß an die Grenzen dieser Maßnahme der Verhaltensprävention. Maßnahmen der Verhältnisprävention, wie die Verkleinerung der Gruppengrößen oder die Verbesserung des Personalschlüssels, können auf Einrichtungsebene nur schwer durchgeführt werden. Die Ergebnisse machen aber deutlich, dass Maßnahmen auf der technisch-organisatorischen Ebene in den meisten Einrichtungen nicht voll ausgeschöpft werden. Ein professionelles Lärmschutzkonzept sollte demnach bei der Gestaltung von Kitas, wenn möglich bereits in der Bauphase, als zentrales Element des Arbeits- und Gesundheitsschutzes von Erzieher/-innen umgesetzt werden.

2 Publikationen

Publikation 1

**Muskuloskelettale Beschwerden und Burnout-Risiko bei ErzieherInnen –
Eine Querschnittsstudie**

*Musculoskeletal Symptoms and Risk of Burnout in Child Care Workers -
A Cross-Sectional Study*

Publikation 2

**Der Effekt von Efford-Reward-Imbalance auf die Gesundheit von ErzieherInnen
in Hamburg**

*The Effect of Effort-Reward Imbalance on the Health of Childcare Workers in
Hamburg: A Longitudinal Study*

Publikation 3

**Der Einsatz von persönlichem Gehörschutz (Otoplastik) bei ErzieherInnen –
eine Pilotstudie**

*Use of the Moulded Hearing Protectors by Childcare Workers -
An Interventional Pilot Study*

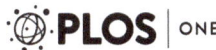

RESEARCH ARTICLE

Musculoskeletal Symptoms and Risk of Burnout in Child Care Workers — A Cross-Sectional Study

Peter Koch[1]*, Johanna Stranzinger[2], Albert Nienhaus[1,2], Agnessa Kozak[1]

1 Centre of Excellence for Epidemiology and Health Services Research for Healthcare Professionals (CVcare), University Medical Centre Hamburg-Eppendorf, Martinistrasse 52, 20246 Hamburg, Germany, **2** Health Protection Division (FBG), Institution for Statutory Accident Insurance and Prevention in the Health and Welfare Services (BGW), Pappelallee 33, 22089 Hamburg, Germany

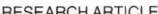

* p.koch@uke.de

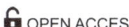

Citation: Koch P, Stranzinger J, Nienhaus A, Kozak A (2015) Musculoskeletal Symptoms and Risk of Burnout in Child Care Workers — A Cross-Sectional Study. PLoS ONE 10(10): e0140980. doi:10.1371/journal.pone.0140980

Editor: Chandrasekharan Nair Kesavachandran, CSIR-Indian Institute of Toxicology Research, INDIA

Received: August 17, 2015

Accepted: October 2, 2015

Published: October 21, 2015

Data Availability Statement: All relevant data are within the paper and its Supporting Information files.

Funding: The authors have no support or funding to report.

Competing Interests: The authors have declared that no competing interests exist.

Abbreviations: ERI, effort reward imbalance; MS, musculoskeletal symptoms; OR, odds ratio; OVC, overcommitment; SD, standard deviation; 95%-CI, 95% confidence interval.

Abstract

Objectives

German child care workers' job satisfaction is influenced by the consequences of unfavourable underlying conditions. Child care workers tend to suffer from psychosocial stress, as they feel that their work is undervalued. The objective of the present study is to investigate how the psychosocial factors of the effort-reward imbalance (ERI) model influence musculoskeletal symptoms (MS) and the risk of burnout. To our knowledge this is the first study investigating the association between the factors of the ERI model and MS in child care workers.

Methods and Findings

Data from 199 child care workers were examined in a cross-sectional study. Psychosocial factors were recorded with the ERI questionnaire. MS was recorded with the Nordic Questionnaire and risk of burnout with the *Personal Burnout* scale of the Copenhagen Burnout Inventory. Multivariate analysis was performed using linear and logistic regression models. The response rate was 57%. In most of the sample (65%), an effort-reward imbalance was observed. 56% of the child care workers were at risk of burnout and 58% reported MS. Factors associated with risk of burnout were *subjective noise exposure* (OR: 4.4, 95%CI: 1.55–12.29) and *overcommitment* (OR: 3.4; 95%CI: 1.46–7.75). There were statistically significant associations between MS and *overcommitment* (low back pain—OR: 2.2, 95%CI: 1.04–4.51), *low control* (overall MS OR: 3.8; 95%CI: 1.68–3.37) and *risk of burnout* (overall MS OR: 2.3, 95%CI: 1.01–5.28). For *ERI* no statistically significant associations were found with reference to risk of burnout or MS.

Conclusion

Overcommitment in child care workers is related to MS and risk of burnout. There is also evidence that *low control* is associated with MS and *subjective noise exposure* with risk of

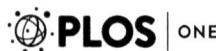

burnout. *Effort-reward imbalance* is not related to either outcome. This occupational health risk assessment identifies changeable working factors in different types of facilities.

Introduction

Burnout is a common phenomenon among employees in the service sector [1]. The occupational group of child care workers is no exception to this—either in Germany or elsewhere [2–6]. Studies in Germany have shown that 10–30% of this occupational group exhibit burnout symptoms or are at risk of burnout [7–9]. Factors associated with burnout in this group include low income, lack of recognition [10, 11] and high noise exposure [12–14]. Low work-associated resources are also associated with burnout. Studies have shown that low control is associated with higher degrees of burnout [15, 16]. The psychosocial situation of employees can be recorded using the factors of the effort-reward imbalance model (ERI model). In the ERI model [17], employee health is related to performance and reward. If there is imbalance between these factors, a stress situation arises (ERI) and the risk of stress-associated diseases increases. Recent German studies have found ERI prevalence values of between 64% and 67% in child care workers [18, 19]. In child care workers and teachers, ERI is strongly correlated with burnout [16]. Overcommitment is a personality trait in the ERI model and is also associated with the risk of burnout in several occupations [20].

International studies have found that child care workers are at increased risk of musculoskeletal symptoms (MS) [8, 21–23]. Both biomechanical and psychosocial factors play a role in the development of MS. Longitudinal studies in several occupational groups have found relevant associations between effort-reward imbalance and MS [24–26]. On the other hand, a review of the association between ERI and MS in all occupations concluded that this association was inconsistent [27]. To our knowledge there have been no studies on this association in child care workers to date.

The primary objective of the present study is to investigate the effect of ERI on MS in child care workers, after allowing for physical stress. The secondary objective is to identify the factors related to the risk of burnout in child care workers.

Material and Methods

As part of occupational risk assessment, a funding provider for facilities for children and adolescents in Hamburg carried out continuous stress monitoring in September 2014. In this study we present the results of a cross-sectional analysis; a follow-up is planned for 2015.

The funding provider bears the responsibility for caring for children in three different types of facility:

1. Day-care centres for children, in which care is provided to children aged up to 6 years.

2. School co-operations: School children in full-time schools are cared for during the afternoon, when there is no teaching.

3. Facilities to support children and adolescents: these include sheltered housing groups and projects for adolescents.

A questionnaire was developed for monitoring and was distributed to 400 employees in 26 different facilities of the funding provider, in collaboration with the works council. Bearing in mind the subsequent follow-up, the questionnaire was performed in a pseudo-anonymous

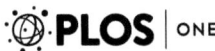 ONE

form. The study was agreed with the data safety officer of the funding provider. The Hamburg Ethics Committee specifically approved this study (reference number: PV4792). Written informed consent was given by all participants.

All employees who worked for at least ten hours per week were invited to take part in the study. In order to reach employees who were on leave at the time of data collection, or who were often absent for other reasons, the participants were allowed four weeks to complete and return the questionnaires.

Aside from demographic information, the questionnaire included information on area of work, weekly working hours, period of employment, everyday working life situations, physical stress, subjective noise exposure, psychosocial factors and work-related resources. The outcomes of risk of burnout and MS were ascertained.

Physical stress, such as lifting or carrying children, was ascertained with selected questions in a validated instrument [28]. A cumulative score could then be calculated from five items (values 5–20), and this records physical stress with respect to *awkward body postures, standing, sitting, and lifting and carrying children. As a predictor this score* was then coded into three different degrees, using the tertile boundaries.

Subjective noise exposure was assessed with 13 questions we had developed ourselves. Items such as: "This level of noise bothers me" or "There are rooms where I hear particularly poorly" were answered on a 5-point scale, ranging from *strongly agree* to *strongly disagree*. A cumulative score was calculated from the answers. The values of the score lied between 13 and 65 points. This variable was classified by the tertile boundaries.

Psychosocial factors were ascertained with the effort-reward imbalance questionnaire (23-Item version) [29]. The psychosocial situation (ERI) and the personality trait of *overcommitment (OVC)* were recorded with 3 scales (*effort*: 6 Items, *reward*: 11 Items and *OVC*: 6 Items). In accordance with the definition, the ERI ratio score was calculated from the ratio of the cumulative scale for *effort* to the cumulative scale for *reward*, with a correction for the different number of items in the two scales: Σ Effort/ΣReward*0.5454. An effort-reward imbalance is defined as an ERI ratio score greater than unity. Independently of the scale range, increased *overcommitment* was defined as a value in the upper tertile of the distribution (third tertile: 16.6).

Other workplace-related stresses and resources were recorded with selected dimensions of a standardised short questionnaire for job analysis [30]. These include *qualitative workload, control, collaboration, information* and *employee participation, integration* and *variety*. All dimensions consisted of several individual items, with a response scale from 1 to 5.

The dimension *Personal Burnout* of the Copenhagen Burnout Inventory [31] served to record the employees' risk of burnout. This scale ranges from 0 to 100: values above 50 are defined as indicating an increased risk of burnout.

Musculoskeletal symptoms (MS) in the shoulder, of the neck and the lower back were recorded with the Nordic Questionnaire [32]. Pain prevalence values were defined by the presence of pain on 8 to 30 days during the previous 12 months *as well as* pain during the 7 days preceding the day of the survey. By combining these two criteria, we hoped to improve the detection of recurrent or persistent pain in these regions of the body.

Statistical Evaluation

The statistical evaluation excluded persons who did not work in child care (e.g. housekeepers or cooks). Group comparisons of normally distributed data were compared with single factor variance analysis. The Kruskal-Wallis test was used as non-parametric test. For bivariate associations between factors and MS (primary research question), odds ratios were calculated from

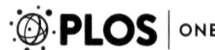 ONE

contingency tables. Logistic regression was used for multivariate analysis. The Hosmer and Lemeshow method was used [33]. This employs a stepwise backwards procedure. Variables with p> 0.1 were successively excluded.

For the second research question, bivariate correlations were calculated with the Spearman correlation coefficient. For multivariate analyses, logistic and linear regressions were calculated with the stepwise backwards procedure. For both research questions, the following variables were included in the regression procedure: *work-related resources, everyday situations at work, ERI, OVC, subjective noise exposure, physical stress, weekly working hours, type of institution, working area, physical activity, age, BMI* and *gender*.

For the variables *ERI* and *OVC*, the models included tests for interactions.

For scales calculated from at least six items the values of the missing items were replaced by the mean value of the available items. If more than half of the individual values of a scale were missing for a participant, the whole scale value was recorded as being missing.

The statistical calculations were performed with the statistics software SPSS Version 22.

Results

Two hundred and thirty of the 400 employees contacted returned the questionnaires (response rate: 57%). Seventeen employees who worked less than ten hours a week and 14 persons working as housekeepers or cooks were subsequently excluded. Thus the data from 199 employees were included in the analysis.

Table 1 describes the characteristics of the employees. The participants in the survey were predominantly women (86.4%). The most frequent age group was between 40 and 50 (29.6%). The mean age was 40 years (not included in the Table). More than 90% were German. 40.2% of the participants had a BMI of at least 25 and 45.7% reported regular physical activity. Almost half (48.7%) worked full-time. Only a few (13.1%) worked in management or administration, but the rest exclusively in child care (86.9%). 56.3% of the participants worked in child day care centres; 26.6% worked in school co-operations and a small proportion (10.6%) in facilities for child and adolescent support. The years of employment could not be evaluated as too many values were missing.

The frequency of situations in typical everyday working life are listed by frequency in Table 2. Many (88.7%) of the participants reported that the situation at work was very noisy; this was most frequent in child day care centres (93.8%). The second most common problem was that the participants felt that the groups were too large (77.5%). The problem with screaming children was most often reported by employees in child day care centres (80.4%). More than half the participants (58.1%) reported that they regularly had conflicts with parents. This was least common for employees in child and adolescent support. Conflicts with colleagues were most frequently given by employees in child day care centres (59.8%). Inadequate breaks were given by 50% and conflicts with management are given by 31.7% of participants.

Table 3 shows the mean values for the different resources and stress scales. For the whole group, the values of the resources were always about 75% of the maximal possible values. The employees of child and adolescent support generally exhibited the highest means. There were statistically significant differences in physical stress and subjective exposure to noise; the employees in child day care exhibited the highest stress levels.

The prevalence of ERI was 65% (mean: 1.17, SD: 0.37) for the whole group. On the other hand, OVC was less prevalent, with 35% (Fig 1). ERI prevalence was greatest for employees in child day care centres (74%). OVC was most frequent in employees of school co-operations (38%).

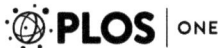

Table 1. Description of the sample.

Variable	N	Percentage
Gender		
Female	172	86.4%
Male	26	13.1%
Missing	1	0.5%
Age in years		
18–30	46	23.1%
30–40	51	25.6%
40–50	59	29.6%
50+	41	20.6%
Missing	2	1.0%
Nationality		
German	184	92.5%
Other	15	7.5%
Missing	0	0.0%
BMI		
>25	115	57.8%
≥25	80	40.2%
Missing	4	2.0%
Physical activity		
Regular	91	45.7%
None	108	54.3%
Missing	0	0.0%
Weekly working hours		
Full-time	97	48.7%
Part-time	102	51.3%
Missing	0	0.0%
Working area		
Management/Administration	26	13.1%
Child Care	173	86.9%
Missing	0	0.0%
Institution		
Child Day Care Centre	112	56.3%
School Co-operation	53	26.6%
Child and Adolescent Support	21	10.6%
Missing	13	6.5%
Total	**199**	**100.0%**

doi:10.1371/journal.pone.0140980.t001

Persons with increased OVC more often exhibited an ERI ratio score above unity in comparison to persons with low OVC (87% vs. 55%) (data not shown in Fig 1). This difference was statistically significant. According to this, approx. 30% of the overall group exhibited increased OVC and ERI at the same time.

Risk of Burnout

A risk of burnout (mean: 51.7, SD: 18.2) was observed for most of the sample (56.8%). The risk of burnout was greatest (64.9%) for employees in child care centres (mean: 54.8, SD: 18.3).

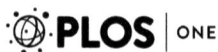

Table 2. Descriptions of situations in everyday working life.

Situation	Child Day Care Centres		School Co-operations		Child and Adolescent Support		Total	
	%	N	%	N	%	N	%	N
It is often too loud where I work.[a]	93.8%	105	86.8%	46	66.7%	14	88.7%	165
Our groups are too large.	79.4%	85	80.4%	41	60%	12	77.5%	138
There are children who suddenly start screaming and cannot be influenced.	80.4%	86	71.7%	38	57.1%	12	75.1%	136
There are conflicts with parents.	60.7%	68	60.4%	32	38.1%	8	58.1%	108
There are conflicts with colleagues.[a]	59.8%	67	41.5%	22	28.6%	6	51.1%	95
Breaks are inadequate.	42.7%	47	60.4%	32	61.9%	13	50.0%	92
There are conflicts with management.	35.8%	39	22.6%	12	33.3%	7	31.7%	58
Total	100%	112	100%	53	100%	21	100%	186

[a]: $p < 0.01$

doi:10.1371/journal.pone.0140980.t002

Correlations were calculated between the continuous factors and the risk of burnout score. The highest statistically significant correlations were found for *OVC* (r = 0.49), *subjective noise exposure* (r = 0.49) and the *ERI ratio score* (r = 0.45). Weaker correlations were found for *effort score* (r = 0.42), *reward score* (r = -0.38), *information and employee participation* (r = -0.35), *qualitative workload* (r = 0.35) and *physical stress* (r = 0.32).

To fulfil the precondition for the linear regression procedure, the ERI variable had to be converted to logarithms. Table 4 shows the standardised beta coefficients and the significances of the final model. *Subjective noise exposure* (beta: 0.315, p: 0.001), *OVC score* (beta: 0.212, p: 0.006) and *qualitative workload* (beta: 0.145, p: 0.044) showed statistically significant relationship to burnout. The logarithm of the *ERI ratio score* exhibited no relevant influence on the outcome (beta: 0.083, p: 0.304).

Table 5 presents the results of the multivariate logistic regression. For persons with increased *OVC*, there was a statistically significant increased risk of burnout (OR: 3.4; 95%CI: 1.46–7.75). However an increase in *ERI* ≥1 had no relevant effect (OR: 1.2; 95%CI: 0.54–2.70). There was a trend in the risk estimates for *subjective noise exposure*. For persons with subjective noise exposure in the third tertile, there was a statistically significant risk increase (OR: 4.4; 95%CI: 1.55–12.29). No statistically significant interaction effect between *ERI* and *OVC* was found in any regression model. The logistic regression model was also calculated using an ERI

Table 3. Resources and stresses in the institutions.

Resource/Stress	Total		Child Day Care Centres	School Co-operations	Child and Adolescent Support	
	$\bar{x}$	SD	$\bar{x}$	$\bar{x}$	$\bar{x}$	P
Control (Scale: 1–5)	3.7	.84	3.8	3.3	3.8	0.001
Variety (Scale: 1–5)	3.8	.76	3.8	3.7	4.3	0.004
Integration (Scale: 1–5)	3.7	.75	3.8	3.5	3.8	0.034
Collaboration (Scale: 1–5)	3.7	.66	3.7	3.5	4.1	0.003
Information and Employee Participation (Scale: 1–5)	3.8	.72	3.8	3.8	3.9	0.907
Qualitative Workload(Scale: 1–5)	2.3	.78	2.3	2.1	2.4	0.093
Physical Stress(Scale: 5–20)	14.2	2.7	15.2	12.5	13.1	0.001
Subjective Noise Exposure (Scale: 13–65)	39	10.3	41	37	32	0.001

doi:10.1371/journal.pone.0140980.t003

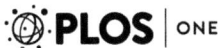
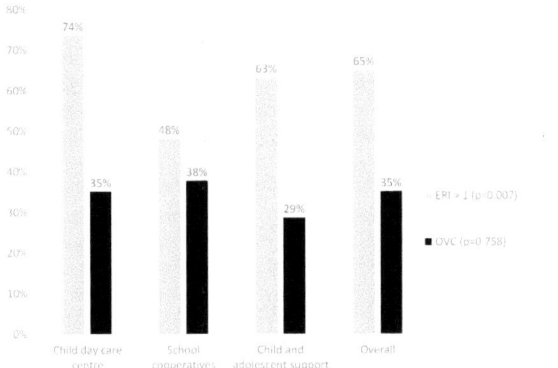

Fig 1. Distribution of the ERI components in the different institutions.

doi:10.1371/journal.pone.0140980.g001

variable with the highest tertile as cut-off point. No statistically significant increase was found in the odds ratio.

Musculoskeletal Symptoms

Fig 2 shows the prevalence for chronic or recurrent MS. Pain in the lower back was most often reported (40%), followed by pain of the neck (35%) and shoulder (16%). The highest prevalence for lower back and shoulder pain were reported for child day care centres (46% or 17%, respectively). The greatest value for neck pain were found for employees of school co-operations (48%).

Table 6 shows the results of the multivariate logistic regression. For the outcome of low back pain, there was a statistically significant increased odds ratio for *OVC* of 2.2 (95%CI: 1.04–4.51). For the outcome of shoulder pain, there was a statistically significant increased odds ratio for *low control* (OR: 3.5; 95%CI: 1.31–9.27). For the neck pain, there were statistically significant increased odds ratios for both *low control* (OR: 4.3; 95%CI: 2.02–9.10) and *risk of burnout* (OR: 2.7; 95%CI: 1.16–6.08).

For the outcome of overall prevalence of MS, there were statistically significant increased odds ratios for *low control* (OR: 3.8, 95%CI: 1.68–3.37), *management* (OR: 4.5, 95%CI: 1.06–

Table 4. Results of the linear regression for the outcome risk of burnout.

	Beta Coefficient [a]	p
Qualitative Workload	0.145	0.044
Subjective Noise Exposure	0.315	0.001
Weekly Working Hours	0.132	0.057
Groups too large	0.125	0.063
ERI Ratio Log Score	0.083	0.304
OVC Score	0.212	0.006

[a]: Standardised beta coefficient adjusted for age, gender and institution, R^2: 0.425

doi:10.1371/journal.pone.0140980.t004

Publikation 1

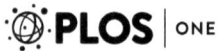
Table 5. Results of the multivariate logistic regression for risk of burnout.

Variable	Specification	OR	95%-CI	p
Variety	High	1	.	.
	Little	2.1	0.98–4.32	0.055
Subjective Noise Exposure	1.Tertile	1	.	.
	2.Tertile	1.9	0.78–4.83	0.150
	3.Tertile	4.4	1.55–12.29	0.005
Physical Stress	1.Tertile	1	.	.
	2.Tertile	1.2	0.37–3.84	0.770
	3.Tertile	2.3	0.97–5.50	0.058
Weekly Working Hours	Part time	1	.	.
	Full time	1.9	0.85–4.43	0.118
ERI	< 1	1	.	.
	≥ 1	1.2	0.54–2.70	0.649
OVC	1./2.Tertile	1	.	.
	3.Tertile	3.4	1.46–7.75	0.004

doi:10.1371/journal.pone.0140980.t005

19.28), *screaming children* (OR: 2.7, 95%CI: 1.01–7.21), as well as for persons at *risk of burnout* (OR: 2.3, 95%CI: 1.10–5.28).

No statistically significant interaction effects between *ERI* and *OVC* were found in any regression model. All models were also calculated with an ERI variable with the highest tertile as cut-off point. Here too no statistically significant increases were found in the odds ratios.

Discussion

Factors such as subjective noise, qualitative workload and OVC showed significant relationships to risk of personal burnout in child care workers.

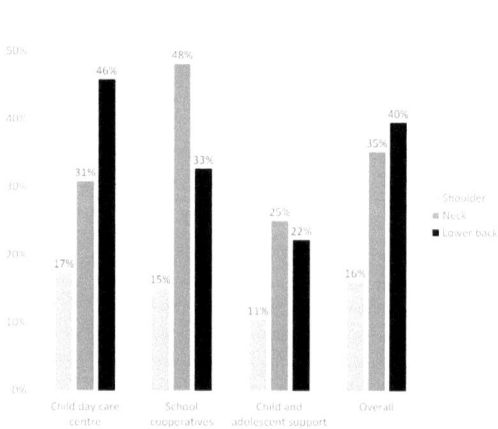

Fig 2. Prevalence of musculoskeletal symptoms.

doi:10.1371/journal.pone.0140980.g002

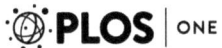

Table 6. Final models of multivariate logistic regression for MS.

Variable	Low Back		Shoulder		Neck		Total MS	
	76 (40%)		32 (16%)		68 (35%)		107 (59%)	
	OR 95% CI	p	OR 95% CI	p	OR 95% CI	p	OR 95% CI	p
Low Control	—		3.5 (1.31–9.27)	0.012	4.3 (2.02–9.10)	0.001	3.8 (1.68–3.37)	0.001
ERI ≥1	1.0 (0.46–2.17)	0.991	0.7 (0.23–1.89)	0.447	0.8 (0.35–1.86)	0.629	0.8 (0.35–1.92)	0.663
OVC Highest Tertile	2.2 (1.04–4.51)	0.038	1.0 (0.36–2.56)	0.953	0.8 (0.35–1.71)	0.537	1.0 (0.43–2.31)	0.998
Working Area: Management vs. Child Care Area	—		—		—		4.5 (1.06–19.28)	0.041
Screaming Children	—		—		—		2.7 (1.01–7.21)	0.047
Risk of Burnout	2.0 (0.96–4.25)	0.063	—		2.7 (1.16–6.08)	0.021	2.3 (1.01–5.28)	0.046

doi:10.1371/journal.pone.0140980.t006

We found significant associations between low control at work and pain in shoulder, neck and total MS. Risk of burnout was associated with neck pain and total MS. For persons with *ERI ratio score > 1* no statistically significant increase in the odds ratios in any region of the body or for risk of burnout were found.

Effort-Reward Imbalance

Nübling et al. [20] observed a mean ERI ratio score of 0.6 for the social professions. We found a mean of 1.17 for child care workers, with a prevalence of 65% for an ERI ratio score > 1 —a comparatively high value. In an older study with child care workers, Scheuch & Seibt [16] also found a lower mean value of 0.5. On the other hand, some current German studies have also found high prevalence values for ERI, including 64% and 67% for teachers and 87% for managers of child care workers [18, 19]. These high prevalence values for ERI could possibly be the result of the expansion of child care within Germany in the past few years, resulting in excessively large groups of children and short term employment contracts. This can, for example, lead to high exposure to noise and more frequent conflict situations in everyday working life.

Musculoskeletal Symptoms

In the context of the present study, no association was found between *ERI ratio score >1* and MS in child care workers. The analysis corrected for the confounder *physical stress*. Even a more stringent classification of ERI by splitting into tertiles [34–36] did not lead to any relevant effects in this study. The observed association between *OVC* and low back pain has been demonstrated in the literature. Bernard et al. [37] found relevant effects in vineyard workers and von der Knesebeck et al. [38] in policemen. Moreover, other studies have found statistically significant associations between *OVC* and MS in other body regions [35, 39–41].

The observed effects for *low control* and shoulder pain, neck pain and total MS are consistent with two reviews. These summarised longitudinal studies and also found associations for pain in the back, neck, shoulder and upper extremities [42, 43]. The demand-control model [44] defines *high demands* and *low control* as unfavourable psychosocial factors. The statistically significant associations with *low control* found in the present study are in contrast with the lack of associations with the psychosocial factors of the ERI model. Excluding *low control* from the multivariate model had only a minimal effect on the odds ratios for *ERI* and *OVC*. In the present study, the dimension *control* was not recorded with the original demand-control questionnaire [30]. Nevertheless we found that the proxy variable *control* is evidently associated with MS, as it records a psychosocial factor that is not included in the ERI model. There is

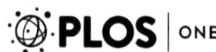

already published evidence that the psychosocial factors in the ERI model and those in the demand-control model are complementary [45, 46].

Persons at *risk of burnout* showed higher odds in neck pain and total MS. Burnout lies at the end of the chain of stress and represents a state proceeded by permanent exposure to stress. It is possible that the scale *Personal Burnout* in the present study more specifically identifies the persons exposed to long-term occupational stress factors and who are therefore at increased risk of MS. The association between burnout and MS has been described in longitudinal and cross-sectional studies [47–49]. Armon et al. [47] and Melamed [48] found statistically signifi-cant effects in white collar workers and in factory workers respectively in longitudinal studies. Kozak et al. [49] described the statistically significant association between burnout and MS in a cross-sectional study in veterinarians.

An increased odds ratio of 4.5 was found for *managers*. This effect is difficult to interpret, as managers tend to work in offices and only rarely have to sit in awkward postures in chairs intended for children. It may be that managerial work is associated with other psychosocial or organisational stress that is linked to MS, but which was not recorded separately.

Risk of Burnout

In a summary of burnout research [1], burnout is described as "a well documented phenome-non in the service provision sector". In the present study we found a considerably high risk of burnout ($\geq$ 50 points: 57%, $\bar{x}$: 52). Reference data for 2013 from the COPSOQ Database give a mean value of 48 for child care workers (data in S1 Supporting Information). Buch & Frieling [8] give the risk of burnout of German child care workers as 30%.

The effects observed in linear regression were confirmed in logistic regression in two of three cases (*OVC* and *subjective noise exposure*).

The statistically significant association between *OVC* and risk of burnout (OR: 3.4) has been observed in managerial staff [40] and also across the different occupational groups [20]. This association has also been demonstrated in health service employees and in teachers [50, 51]. It seems plausible that an underlying attendance for excessive working is a premise for the devel-opment of burnout symptoms.

In the present study, *subjective noise exposure* was not recorded with a validated instrument, but with a questionnaire specially developed for this setting. Nevertheless, the observed associa-tion with risk of burnout appears to be reliable; in both regression procedures, *subjective noise exposure* exhibits the greatest effect estimates in the model. The evidence for a trend in the risk estimates in the logistic regression model also supports a robust association with the burnout risk. Child care workers are exposed to a special sort of noise. Studies have shown that loud speech requires more attention and cognitive effort than meaningless noise, e.g. noise from machines [52]. This also applies when the information content of the speech is irrelevant for the listeners. In the present study, 77% of participants reported that the groups were too large and 88% that it was often too loud. We assume that there is massive stress from this type of noise. Other studies in child care workers report mean individual noise levels between 71 and 83 db(A) on one working day, maximum levels reaching levels above 100 db(A) [12–14]. Although our study does not assess objective noise levels, the correlation between subjective noise perception und measured individual noise levels is known [53].

For child care workers and teachers an association between subjective or objective noise and burnout has been observed elsewhere [12, 54]. Sjodin et al. [12] conclude that subjective noise exposure does not contribute do the development of burnout. Furthermore this association shows that workers with an elevated risk of burnout tend to develop an increased sensitivity to noise. Therefore they are more vulnerable to noise. However, known adverse health effects due

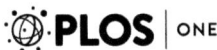

to noise exposure are coronary heart disease, hypertension, stress and sleep disturbance [55–58]. In the context of day care centres high noise levels may cause auditory fatigue [59]. Furthermore, from the children's view continuous noise levels reduce intelligibility and verbal acquisition amongst children in classrooms [60]. This report assumes the results of an occupational health risk assessment. However, children's health is at least just as important in this setting, but not the focus of this paper.

The dimension of *qualitative workload* employs two items to record the concentration required and the complexity of the work. The observed—albeit low—association with risk of burnout shows the challenges of having to concentrate. Potentially this association can also be explained by an inverse causality: child care workers with increased risk of burnout experience a major challenge performing work tasks that require high levels of concentration, e.g. listening to informative noise.

In general, strikingly high prevalence values were found in this study, particularly ERI, OVC, risk of burnout, MS and situations in everyday working life. The responses may have been influenced by current changes in the occupational situation of child care workers in Germany. The results may have been biased by long-term dissatisfaction at work, the wish to change the underlying conditions, as well as social desirability. It is possible that the results would have been similar for another sample from another location in Germany at the same point in time.

Limitations

The response rate was 57%, which was a relatively good value for a group of employees. However, a non-responder analysis was not performed, so it is not possible to conclude whether the missing group of persons was distinct from the sample in any way.

Due to the cross-sectional design, it is not possible to establish causality. It is theoretically possible that the direction of the causality is the opposite of what we have assumed. A longitudinal study has demonstrated that MS is a predictor of effort-reward imbalance [61]. A bias from common-method variance is likely, e.g. from social desirability [62]. Concededly no objective noise measures were performed in this study. Subjective noise exposure, however, was detected as a relevant factor.

Work-related psychosocial factors are a part of working life. We did not control for the effect of psychosocial factors on private life, e.g. stress in the family. We also failed to consider other factors in the overall psychosocial situation of the employees that complement the factors in the ERI model. For example, these include the entire components of the job demand-control model [44]. Moreover, the odds ratios in this study are overestimated. As the prevalence values of the outcome variables are high, the risk estimates must be interpreted with caution.

Conclusion

The study results provide risk assessments that permits the inference of specific objectives and interventions for workers in different institutions. Workers with a high risk of burnout appear as vulnerable workers. At the level of the individual place of work, objectives should concentrate on noise and the resource control, as both of these factors may influence the well-being and both can be changed. Historically child care workers were not considered to be have a noisy workplace. However, this study provides new results implicating that occupational safety and health protection should be modified accordingly. Suitable measures for reducing noise should be introduced to the workplaces and then evaluated. In addition, the possibilities should be determined of enhancing control in organisation at work. The existing situation should be analysed and possibly reorganised.

Publikation 1

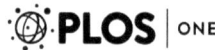 | ONE

Supporting Information

S1 Supporting information. Statement Personal Burnout COPSOQ Database.
(PDF)

Acknowledgments

We thank Dr. Matthias Nübling for assistance with unpublished data of the Copenhagen Psychosocial Questionnaire (COPSOQ) database.

Author Contributions

Conceived and designed the experiments: PK JS. Performed the experiments: PK. Analyzed the data: PK. Contributed reagents/materials/analysis tools: PK AN. Wrote the paper: PK. Was critically reading the manuscript: JS AN AK. Read the draft critically and gave substantial comments for the improvement of the first draft: AN. Revised the manuscript critically for important intellectual content and gave final approval for the version to be published: AK.

References

1. Schaufeli WB, Buunk BP. Burnout: An overview of 25 years of research and theorizing. In: Schabracq MJ, Winnubst JA, Cooper CL, editors. The handbook of work and health psychology. 2nd edn ed. New York: Wiley & Sons; 2003. p. 383–425.
2. Manlove EE. Multiple correlates of burnout in child care workers. Early Childhood Research Quarterly. 1993; 8(4):499–518.
3. Kushnir T, Milbauer V. Managing stress and burnout at work: A cognitive group intervention. Program for directors of day care centers. Meeting the needs of caregivers: Occupational health and safety issues for child care providers. International Conference on Child Day Care Health: Science, Prevention and Practice; June 15–17; Atlanta, USA1992.
4. Whitebook M, Howes C, Darrah R, Friedman J. Who's minding the child care workers? A look at staff burnout. Children Today. 1980; 10(1):2–6.
5. Bertolino B, Thompson K. The residential youth care worker in action. Binghamton, New York: Hawthorn Press; 1999.
6. Snow K. Aggression: Just part of the job? The psychological impact of aggression on child and youth workers. Journal of Child and Youth Care. 1994; 9(4):11–30.
7. Rudow B. Belastungen im Erzieher/innenberuf. Bildung & Wissenschaft. 2004(6:):6–11.
8. Buch M, Frieling E. Belastungs- und Beanspruchungsoptimierung in Kindertagesstätten. Kassel: Eigenverlag Universität Kassel, Institut für Arbeitswissenschaft; 2001.
9. Jungbauer J, Ehlen A. Stressbelastungen und Burnout-Risiko bei Erzieherinnen in Kindertagesstätten. Ergebnisse einer Fragebogenstudie. Gesundheitswesen. 2014.
10. Whitebook M, Howes C, Phillips D. Who cares? Child care teachers and the quality of care in America: Final Report of the National Child Care Staffing Study. Oakland, CA: Child Care Employee Project, 1989.
11. Caring for a Living: A Study on the Wages and Working Conditions in Canadian Child Care. Final Report. Washington, D.C.: Canadian Child Care Federation, Ottawa, 1992.
12. Sjödin F, Kjellberg A, Knutsson A, Landstrom U, Lindberg L. Noise and stress effects on preschool personnel. Noise & health. 2012; 14(59):166–78.
13. Eysel-Gosepath K, Pape HG, Erren T, Thinschmidt M, Lehmacher W, Piekarski C. [Sound levels in nursery schools]. Hno. 2010; 58(10):1013–20. doi: 10.1007/s00106-010-2121-y PMID: 20480127
14. Paulsen R. Noise Exposure in Kindergartens. In: Akustik DGf, editor. CFA/DAGA'04 30 Jahrestagung für Akustik—Europäische Akustik-Ausstellung; 22.-25. März; Straßburg2004. p. 573–4.
15. Arches J. Social structure, burnout, and job satisfaction. Social work. 1991; 36(3):202–6. PMID: 2057805
16. Scheuch K, Seibt R. Arbeits- und persönlichkeitsbedingte Beziehungen zu Burnout—eine kritische Betrachtung. In: Richter PG, Rau R, Mühlpfordt S, editors. Arbeit und Gesundheit Lengerich: Pabst Science Publishers; 2007. p. 42–54.

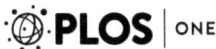 ONE

17. Siegrist J. Adverse health effects of high-effort/low-reward conditions. Journal of occupational health psychology. 1996; 1(1):27–41. PMID: 9547031

18. Schreyer I, Krause M, Brandl M, Nicko O. AQUA Arbeitsplatz und Qualität in Kitas Ergebnisse einer bundesweiten Befragung. München: Staatsinstitut für Frühpädagogik, 2014.

19. Viernickel S, Voss A, Mauz E, Gerstenberg F, Schumann M. STEGE—Strukturqualität und Erzieher_-innengesundheit in Kindertageseinrichtungen. Wissenschaftlicher Abschlussbericht. 2013.

20. Nübling M, Seidler A, Garthus-Niegel S, Latza U, Wagner M, Hegewald J, et al. The Gutenberg Health Study: measuring psychosocial factors at work and predicting health and work-related outcomes with the ERI and the COPSOQ questionnaire. BMC public health. 2013; 13:538. doi: 10.1186/1471-2458-13-538 PMID: 23734632

21. Grant KA, Habes DJ, Tepper AL. Work activities and musculoskeletal complaints among preschool workers. Applied ergonomics. 1995; 26(6):405–10. PMID: 15677041

22. Gratz RR, Claffey A. Adult health in childcare: health status, behaviors, and concerns of teachers, directors, and family child care providers. Early Childhood Research Quarterly. 1996; 11(2):243–67.

23. Botzet M, Frank H. Arbeit und Gesundheit von Mitarbeiterinnen in Kindertageseinrichtungen. Regionalfallstudie in saarländischen Kindertageseinrichtungen. Saarbrücken: Landesarbeitsgemeinschaft für Gesundheitsförderung Saarland e.V., 1998.

24. Rugulies R, Krause N. Effort-reward imbalance and incidence of low back and neck injuries in San Francisco transit operators. Occupational and environmental medicine. 2008; 65(8):525–33. PMID: 18056748

25. Lapointe J, Dionne CE, Brisson C, Montreuil S. Effort-reward imbalance and video display unit postural risk factors interact in women on the incidence of musculoskeletal symptoms. Work. 2013; 44(2):133–43. doi: 10.3233/WOR-2012-1357 PMID: 22927580

26. Krause N, Burgel B, Rempel D. Effort-reward imbalance and one-year change in neck-shoulder and upper extremity pain among call center computer operators. Scandinavian journal of work, environment & health. 2010; 36(1):42–53.

27. Koch P, Schablon A, Latza U, Nienhaus A. Musculoskeletal pain and effort-reward imbalance—a systematic review. BMC public health. 2014; 14:37. doi: 10.1186/1471-2458-14-37 PMID: 24428955

28. Slesina W. FEBA: Fragebogen zur subjektiven Einschätzung der Belastungen am Arbeitsplatz. ASER-Institut: wwwrueckenkompassde2009.

29. Siegrist J, Starke D, Chandola T, Godin I, Marmot M, Niedhammer I, et al. The measurement of effort-reward imbalance at work: European comparisons. Social science & medicine. 2004; 58(8):1483–99.

30. Prümper J, Hartmannsgruber K, Frese M. KFZA—Kurzfragebogen zur Arbeitsanalyse. Zeitschrift für Arbeits- und Organisationspsychologie. 1995; 39(3):125–32.

31. Kristensen TS, Hannerz H, Hogh A, Borg V. The Copenhagen Psychosocial Questionnaire—a tool for the assessment and improvement of the psychosocial work environment. Scandinavian journal of work, environment & health. 2005; 31(6):438–49.

32. Kuorinka I, Jonsson B, Kilbom A, Vinterberg H, Biering-Sorensen F, Andersson G, et al. Standardised Nordic questionnaires for the analysis of musculoskeletal symptoms. Applied ergonomics. 1987; 18 (3):233–7. PMID: 15676628

33. Hosmer DW, Lemeshow S. Applied logistic regression. New York: Wiley & Sons; 2000.

34. Weyers S, Peter R, Boggild H, Jeppesen HJ, Siegrist J. Psychosocial work stress is associated with poor self-rated health in Danish nurses: a test of the effort-reward imbalance model. Scandinavian journal of caring sciences. 2006; 20(1):26–34. PMID: 16489957

35. Dragano N, von dem Knesebeck O, Rodel A, Siegrist J. Psychosoziale Arbeitsbelastungen und muskuloskeletale Beschwerden: Bedeutung für die Prävention. Journal of Public Health. 2003; 11(3):196–207.

36. de Jonge J, Bosma H, Peter R, Siegrist J. Job strain, effort-reward imbalance and employee well-being: a large-scale cross-sectional study. Social science & medicine. 2000; 50(9):1317–27.

37. Bernard C, Courouve L, Bouée S, Adjémian A, Chrétien JC, Niedhammer I. Biomechanical and psychosocial work exposures and musculoskeletal symtoms among vineyard workers. Journal of Occupational Health. 2011; 53(5):297–311. PMID: 21778662

38. von dem Knesebeck O, David K, Siegrist J. [Psychosocial stress at work and musculoskeletal pain among police officers in special forces]. Gesundheitswesen. 2005; 67(8–9):674–9. PMID: 16217722

39. Tsutsumi A, Shitake T, Peter R, Siegrist S, Matoba T. The Japanese version of the Efford-Reward Imbalance Questionnaire: a study in dental technicians. Work & Stress. 2001b; 15(1):86–96.

40. Lau B. Effort-reward imbalance and overcommitment in employees in a Norwegian municipality: a cross sectional study. Journal of occupational medicine and toxicology. 2008; 3:9. doi: 10.1186/1745-6673-3-9 PMID: 18447923

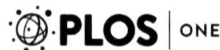 | ONE

41. Joksimovic L, Starke D, v d Knesebeck O, Siegrist J. Perceived work stress, overcommitment, and self-reported musculoskeletal pain: a cross-sectional investigation. International journal of behavioral medicine. 2002; 9(2):122–38. PMID: 12174531

42. Kraatz S, Lang J, Kraus T, Munster E, Ochsmann E. The incremental effect of psychosocial workplace factors on the development of neck and shoulder disorders: a systematic review of longitudinal studies. International archives of occupational and environmental health. 2013; 86(4):375–95. doi: 10.1007/s00420-013-0848-y PMID: 23549669

43. Lang J, Ochsmann E, Kraus T, Lang JW. Psychosocial work stressors as antecedents of musculoskeletal problems: a systematic review and meta-analysis of stability-adjusted longitudinal studies. Social science & medicine. 2012; 75(7):1163–74.

44. Karasek RA. Job Demands, Job Decision Latitude, and Mental Strain: Implications for Job Redesign. Administrative Science Quarterly. 1979; 24(2):285–308.

45. Tsutsumi A, Kayaba K, Theorell T, Siegrist J. Association between job stress and depression among Japanese employees threatened by job loss in a comparison between two complementary job-stress models. Scandinavian journal of work, environment & health. 2001a; 27(2):146–53.

46. Bosma H, Peter R, Siegrist J, Marmot M. Two alternative job stress models and the risk of coronary heart disease. American journal of public health. 1998; 88(1):68–74. PMID: 9584036

47. Armon G, Melamed S, Shirom A, Shapira I. Elevated burnout predicts the onset of musculoskeletal pain among apparently healthy employees. Journal of occupational health psychology. 2010; 15 (4):399–408. doi: 10.1037/a0020726 PMID: 21058854

48. Melamed S. Burnout and risk of regional musculoskeletal pain—A prospective study of apparently healthy employed adults. Stress & Health. 2009; 25(4):313–21.

49. Kozak A, Schedlbauer G, Peters C, Nienhaus A. Self-reported musculoskeletal disorders of the distal upper extremities and the neck in German veterinarians: a cross-sectional study. PloS one. 2014; 9(2): e89362. doi: 10.1371/journal.pone.0089362 PMID: 24586718

50. Wang Y, Ramos A, Wu H, Liu L, Yang X, Wang J, et al. Relationship between occupational stress and burnout among Chinese teachers: a cross-sectional survey in Liaoning, China. International archives of occupational and environmental health. 2015; 88(5):589–97. doi: 10.1007/s00420-014-0987-9 PMID: 25256806

51. Chou LP, Li CY, Hu SC. Job stress and burnout in hospital employees: comparisons of different medical professions in a regional hospital in Taiwan. BMJ open. 2014; 4(2):e004185. doi: 10.1136/bmjopen-2013-004185 PMID: 24568961

52. Venetjoki N, Kaarlela-Tuomaala A, Keskinen E, Hongisto V. The effect of speech and speech intelligibility on task performance. Ergonomics. 2006; 49(11):1068–91. PMID: 16950722

53. Neitzel RL, Svensson EB, Sayler SK, Ann-Christin J. A comparison of occupational and nonoccupational noise exposures in Sweden. Noise & health. 2014; 16(72):270–8.

54. Santana AMC, De Marchi D, Junior LCG, Girondoli YM, Chiappete A. Burnout syndrome, working conditions, and health: a reality among public high school teachers in Brazil. Work. 2012; 41(S1):3709–17.

55. Gan WQ, Davies HW, Demers PA. Exposure to occupational noise and cardiovascular disease in the United States: the National Health and Nutrition Examination Survey 1999–2004. Occupational and environmental medicine. 2011; 68(3):183–90. doi: 10.1136/oem.2010.055269 PMID: 20924023

56. Bodin T, Albin M, Ardo J, Stroh E, Ostergren PO, Bjork J. Road traffic noise and hypertension: results from a cross-sectional public health survey in southern Sweden. Environmental health: a global access science source. 2009; 8:38.

57. Hebert S, Lupien SJ. Salivary cortisol levels, subjective stress, and tinnitus intensity in tinnitus sufferers during noise exposure in the laboratory. International journal of hygiene and environmental health. 2009; 212(1):37–44. doi: 10.1016/j.ijheh.2007.11.005 PMID: 18243788

58. de Kluizenaar Y, Janssen SA, van Lenthe FJ, Miedema HME, Mackenbach JP. Long-term road traffic noise exposure is associated with an increase in morning tiredness. J Acoust Soc Am. 2009; 126 (2):626–33. doi: 10.1121/1.3158834 PMID: 19640028

59. Truchon-Gagnon C, Hétu R. Noise in day-care centres for children. Noise Control Eng J. 1988; 30:57–64.

60. Picard M, Bradley JS. Revisiting speech interference in classrooms. Audiology: official organ of the International Society of Audiology. 2001; 40(5):221–44.

61. Bonzini M, Bertu L, Veronesi G, Conti M, Coggon D, Ferrario MM. Is musculoskeletal pain a consequence or a cause of occupational stress? A longitudinal study. International archives of occupational and environmental health. 2015; 88(5):607–12. doi: 10.1007/s00420-014-0982-1 PMID: 25261316

62. Podsakoff PM, MacKenzie SB, Lee JY, Podsakoff NP. Common method biases in behavioral research: a critical review of the literature and recommended remedies. The Journal of applied psychology. 2003; 88(5):879–903. PMID: 14516251

Koch et al. Journal of Occupational Medicine and Toxicology (2017) 12:16
DOI 10.1186/s12995-017-0163-8

Journal of Occupational
Medicine and Toxicology

RESEARCH Open Access

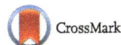

The effect of effort-reward imbalance on the health of childcare workers in Hamburg: a longitudinal study

Peter Koch[1]*, Jan Felix Kersten[1], Johanna Stranzinger[1] and Albert Nienhaus[1,2]

Abstract

Background: The prevalence of effort-reward imbalance (ERI) among qualified childcare workers in Germany is currently estimated at around 65%. High rates of burnout and musculoskeletal symptoms (MS) have also been reported for this group. Previous longitudinal studies show inconsistent results with regard to the association between ERI and MS. As yet, no longitudinal studies have been conducted to investigate the association between ERI and burnout or MS in childcare workers. This study aims to investigate the extent to which a relationship between ERI and MS or burnout can be observed in childcare workers in Germany on a longitudinal basis.

Methods: In 2014 childcare workers ($N = 199$, response rate: 57%) of a provider of facilities for children and youth in Hamburg were asked about stress and health effects in the workplace. Follow-up was completed one year later ($N = 106$, follow-up rate: 53%) For the baseline assessment, ERI was determined as the primary influencing factor. Data on MS was recorded using the Nordic questionnaire, and burnout using the personal burnout scale of the Copenhagen Burnout Inventory (CBI). The statistical analysis was carried out using multivariate linear and logistic regression.

Results: At baseline ERI was present in 65% of the sample population. The mean burnout score at the time of follow-up was 53.7 (SD: 20.7); the prevalence of MS was between 19% and 62%. ERI was identified as a statistically significant factor for MS, after adjusting especially for physical stress (lower back: OR 4.2; 95% CI: 1.14 to 15.50, neck: OR 4.3; 95% CI: 1.25 to 15.0, total MS: OR 4.0; 95% CI: 1.20 to 13.49). With regard to burnout, a relative increase of 10% in the ERI ratio score increased the burnout score by 1.1 points ($p = 0.034$).

Conclusions: ERI was revealed to be a major factor in relation to MS and burnout in childcare workers. Based on this observation worksite interventions on the individual and organizational level should be introduced in order to prevent ERI.

Keywords: Musculoskeletal symptoms, Burnout, Psychosocial, Nursery teacher, Occupational disease, Esteem, Work-related

Background

Current German studies report unfavourable psychosocial working conditions for childcare workers. According to these studies, the prevalence of work-related effort-reward imbalance [1] is in between 64% and 67% [2–4]. In Siegrist's effort-reward imbalance model (ERI model), the health of the employee is associated with performance and rewards (esteem, job security and promotion). The model is based on the assumption that there should ideally be a reciprocal relationship between efforts and socially defined rewards. If rewards are lower than efforts, a stressful situation that increases the risk of stress-related diseases occurs for the employee. Empirical evidence for this hypothesis has been found mainly for coronary heart disease, cardiovascular disease and depression [5]. A special feature of the ERI model is the inclusion of over-commitment (OVC) personality as a personal trait that represents a coping

* Correspondence: p.koch@uke.de
[1]Centre of Excellence for Epidemiology and Health Services Research for
Healthcare Professionals (CVcare), University Medical Centre
Hamburg-Eppendorf, Martinistrasse 52, 20246 Hamburg, Germany
Full list of author information is available at the end of the article

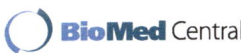

Koch et al. Journal of Occupational Medicine and Toxicology (2017) 12:16

strategy in combination with high demands. OVC generates excessive commitment in conjunction with expectations of high rewards. According to Siegrist employees with OVC are also at increased risk, and in combination with ERI even higher risk, for developing stress-related diseases. Observations in German teachers found that OVC negatively affected plasma co-agulation, natural killer cells and T-helper cells [6, 7]. Furthermore, depression and somatic symptoms including MS were found to be associated with the interaction of OVC and ERI in nurses [8, 9].

International studies have observed an increased risk of musculoskeletal disorders among childcare workers [10–13]. The association between the increase of MS and the factors of the ERI model has been observed in longitudinal studies of employee cohorts in different industries [14–16]. In a systematic review of all industries, however, the association between ERI and MS has been evaluated as inconsistent on the basis of cross-sectional and longitudinal studies [17]. To our knowledge, there have not yet been performed any longitudinal studies examining the association between ERI and MS in childcare workers.

Another symptom associated with stress in the workplace is burnout. Employees working in the service sector show a high risk of burnout [18]. Childcare workers as an occupational group do not represent any exception to this in international comparisons [19–23]. For childcare workers in Germany, prevalence rates of between 10% and 57% have been observed for burnout symptoms [2, 10, 24, 25]. For childcare workers and teaching staff, ERI shows a strong correlation with burnout [26]. A greater tendency towards OVC was shown to be associated with burnout in cross-sectional studies of qualified childcare workers and across industries [2, 27]. Longitudinal studies investigating the association between ERI and burnout in childcare workers have not been published yet.

We aim to address the following research questions in this study:

1. Does a longitudinal approach reveal an association between the psychosocial factors of the ERI model and MS among childcare workers?
2. Does a longitudinal approach reveal an association between the ERI ratio score and a higher risk of burnout among childcare workers?

Methods

As part of a 2014 occupational risk assessment a funding provider for children and young people comprising 26 different facilities in Hamburg carried out a stress monitoring survey of its childcare workers [2]. In this paper the results of the follow-up investigation of this multi-centre study are presented.

In November 2014, all 400 qualified childcare workers of all different facilities were asked about health and stresses they faced at work. A total of 230 questionnaires were returned (response rate: 57%); a total of 31 participants were excluded as a result of low weekly working hours (< 10 h) and employment in domestic/janitorial services (kitchens, workshops). At the time of the baseline assessment, 199 people were therefore included into the study. After twelve months (follow up), all study participants once again received a copy of the same pseudonymised questionnaire they had completed a year before. A subgroup of participants ($n = 33$) took part in a parallel intervention programme looking at the effects of noise in the workplace [28]. In that study, the focus was on the question of whether the use of personal hearing protection over the observational period of one year could reduce the subjective noise exposure and the risk of burnout among childcare workers.

The pseudonymised stress monitoring questionnaire was agreed with the data safety officer of the funding provider for children and young people. Before the study started, every participant gave informed written consent for taking part in the study. All study documents, including the study protocol, were reviewed and approved by the Hamburg Medical Chamber Ethics Committee as part of an application process (reference: PV4792).

Questionnaire

In addition to demographic variables, the questionnaire also collected information on work-related stress and resources. Burnout and MS were used as outcomes.

Physical stress was recorded using selected questions from a standardised questionnaire [29]. Five different types of stress (*awkward body postures, standing, sitting, lifting heavy loads/children* and *carrying heavy loads/children*) were identified on a four-stage frequency scale. This resulted in a corresponding total score (ranging between 5 and 20). Using the median, the variable was dichotomised into the categories of low or high physical stress.

Subjective noise exposure was estimated using a questionnaire developed by the authors. Responding to 13 items on a five-stage scale resulted in a total score (ranging between 13 and 65). This was dichotomised into high and low subjective noise exposure by using the median. For more information, please see the publication of the cross-sectional study [2].

Psychosocial factors were recorded using the ERI questionnaire (23-item version) [30]. The psychosocial situation and the personality trait of *OVC* were evaluated using three scales (*effort*: six items, *reward*: eleven items and *OVC*: six items). The ERI ratio score was determined

Publikation 2

Koch *et al. Journal of Occupational Medicine and Toxicology* (2017) 12:16   Page 3 of 9

according to the definition using a formula that takes into account the different numbers of items in order to calculate the total on the *effort* scale as a ratio to the *reward* scale: Σ Effort/ΣReward*0.5454. An effort-reward imbalance was defined as an ERI ratio score of more than 1. Since this value is not a clinically valid cut-off value, ERI was also tested using the quartile thresholds as an ordinal influencing variable in the analysis. Regardless of the scale, increased *OVC* was defined for the value range in the upper tertile of the empirical distribution and treated as a dichotomous variable.

Other workplace-related characteristics were recorded using selected scales from a standardized instrument, the brief workplace analysis questionnaire (KFZA) [31]. This included both stress factors (*qualitative workload: two items, quantitative workload: two items*) and resources (*control: three items, collaboration: three items, information and employee participation: two items, completeness: two items, variety: three items*). The individual items were rated on a five-stage scale.

In addition, the respondent was asked about the occurrence of typical everyday situations in the workplace. Seven different statements, such as "I experience conflicts with parents" or "I don't get any breaks or chances to step away from work for a while" could be answered with yes or no.

Musculoskeletal symptoms were recorded using the Nordic questionnaire [32]. The prevalence of chronic pain in the shoulder, neck or lower back was defined as the presence of pain on at least eight days in the past twelve months, as well as pain within seven days of filling in the questionnaire. In addition, a comprehensive variable was derived for the presence of at least one type of chronic pain in the three body regions (MS total).

In order to evaluate *burnout* in childcare workers, the *personal burnout* sub-scale from the Copenhagen Burnout Inventory was used [33]. According to the definition, a higher risk of burnout is present with a value of ≥ 50 (range 0–100).

Statistical analysis

For paired group comparisons, the paired t-test was calculated in the case of normally distributed data; for not normally distributed data the Mann–Whitney U test was calculated. For dichotomous paired data, the McNemar test was used. For independent data, the Pearson correlation coefficient was used. In order to evaluate a difference in nominal variables, the chi-squared test was used.

Multivariate logistic regression was calculated for the first research question. Starting with a core variable set (ERI, physical stress, pain T0, participation in intervention programme), all variables with a *p*-value of <0.25 in the bivariate analysis were successively integrated into the model [34]. Physical stress was included as an

important confounder in the relationship between ERI and MS [16]. The following variables were taken into account as potentially influential variables: *work-related resources and stress (KFZA), typical everyday situations in the workplace, subjective noise exposure, physical stress, weekly working hours, type of institution, field of work, physical activity, age, BMI and gender.*

With regard to the second hypothesis, linear regression was used. Starting with a core variable set (ERI, burnout T0, age, participation in a prevention programme, type of institution) all other variables were included that showed a *p*-value of <0.2 in the bivariate analysis. In the second step, the stepwise backwards regression procedure was applied [34], where all variables with *p*-value of >0.1 were excluded from the model. In order to fulfil the requirements of linear regression, the ERI variable was transformed to the logarithmic scaling.

In all multivariate analyses a possible interaction between ERI and OVC was also tested. For logistic regression models a variable with four categories has been built: 1: ERI No/ OVC No, 2: ERI Yes/ OVC No, 3: ERI No/ OVC Yes, 4: ERI Yes/OVC Yes. For linear regression models a multiplicative term has been built from the continuous OVC variable and ERI ratio variable [35].

Missing values were replaced in the ERI scale (effort, reward, OVC) and in the personal burnout scale by individual mean values. If more than half of the individual items on a particular scale were missing for a participant, the entire scale value was set to a missing value.

A dropout analysis was performed using logistic regression. The statistical analysis was carried out using SPSS Statistics, version 23.

Results

At the time of the follow-up, the cohort comprises 106 employees (see Table 1) (Follow-up rate: 53%). The study participants are predominantly women (90.6%). The study participants in the follow-up are statistically significantly older than the dropouts (43 vs 37, *p* < 0.001); age was the only statistically significant variable in the dropout analysis. More than 90% have German nationality. Almost half of the participants have a BMI of ≥ 25 (47%). Overall, 51.9% of the employees report regular physical exercise. More than half (52.8%) work full time, with the majority working exclusively in child care (84.9%). Of all of the employees, 66% are from child day care centres, 21.7% work in school partnerships (caring for school-age children in schools) and the lowest proportion (11.3%) come from child and youth support facilities (youth projects and residential groups). As a result of too many missing values (> 50%), working hours are not evaluated.

Table 2 shows the influential and outcome variables at the time of baseline and follow-up. In terms of

Publikation 2

Koch *et al. Journal of Occupational Medicine and Toxicology* (2017) 12:16

Page 4 of 9

Table 1 Description of the cohort at the time of follow up

Variable	n	Percent
Gender		
Women	96	90.6%
Men	10	9.4%
Age in years		
18–29	16	15.1%
30–39	22	20.8%
40–49	38	35.8%
50+	29	27.4%
n/a	1	0.9%
Nationality		
German	98	92.5%
Other	8	7.5%
BMI		
< 25	54	50.9%
≥ 25	50	47.1%
n/a	2	1.9%
Physical exercise		
Regular	55	51.9%
None	51	48.1%
Area of work		
Child care	90	84.9%
Management/administration	16	15.1%
Weekly working hours		
Full time	56	52.8%
Part time	50	47.2%
Institution		
Child day care centre	70	66%
School partnership	23	21.7%
Child and youth support work	12	11.3%
n/a	1	0.9%
Total	106	100%

resources, the mean values of the variables are ranging between 3.5 and 3.9 at both points in time. This corresponds to an occurrence of 70–78% in the upper end of the scale for individual resources. The mean value for *collaboration* shows a statistically significant decrease over time. Here, the mean decreases from 3.7 to 3.5 ($p = 0.006$). Among the stress factors, there are no statistically significant changes over time for any variables with the exception of ERI. The ERI ratio score increases from 1.2 to 1.3 points ($p < 0.001$), while the difference in the dichotomised ERI variable is also statistically significant (65.1% vs 87.4%, $p < 0.001$). Figure 1 shows which of the ERI sub-scales is mainly responsible for the significant increase in the ERI

ratio score. The mean of the *effort* scale remains nearly constant over time (73 vs. 72). For the three sub-scales of the reward scale, the following trends can be observed: *promotion* increases by three points over time (45 vs 48), *esteem* and *security*, however, decrease statistically significant over time. Here, the mean values decrease from 62 to 49 ($p < 0.001$) and from 67 to 31 ($p < 0.001$) respectively.

With regard to the outcome variables (Table 2), a slight increase in burnout can be observed (50.6 vs 53.7), which is only just not statistically significant ($p = 0.056$). For neck pain (32.1% vs 39.4%), shoulder pain (15.1% vs 19.2%) and MS overall (55.7% vs 62.1%), slight increases can be observed. The prevalence of lower back pain (39.6% vs 34.6%) decreases slightly over time. These differences are not statistically significant.

The results of the multivariate logistic regression of the association between ERI and MS are listed in Table 3. For the outcome of lower back pain, the odds ratio is 4.2 times higher for child care workers with an ERI of >1 (95% CI: 1.14 to 15.50). This correlation is statistically significant. For shoulder pain, an ERI of >1 reveals an increased odds ratio of 1.5 (95% CI: 0.40 to 5.58), which is not statistically significant. In addition, participants with low control show an odds ratio that is 4.5 times higher for shoulder pain (95% CI: 1.15 to 17.42), which is statistically significant. OVC was observed to have a protective effect that was not statistically significant (OR: 0.4; 95% CI: 0.09 to 1.40). With regard to neck pain, an ERI of >1 resulted in a statistically significant higher odds ratio of 4.3 (95% CI: 1.25 to 15.0). For the outcome of total MS, employees with an increased ERI ratio score were also observed to have a statistically significant increase in the odds ratio (OR: 4.0; 95% CI: 1.20 to 13.49). Child care workers who state that they have physical exercise regularly are shown to have a statistically significant protective effect with regard to MS (OR: 0.3; 95% CI: 0.10 to 0.98). Employees who state that they experience conflicts with parents have a statistically significant increase in the risk of MS (OR: 4.9; 95% CI: 1.55 to 15.75). No interaction between ERI and OVC was observed in any of the models.

With regard to burnout, it is shown that the ERI ratio score has a statistically significant influence on increasing the risk of burnout. Translated to the delogrithmed scaling, an increase in the ERI ratio score of 10% would increase the burnout value by 1.1 points (95% CI: 0.09 to 2.14) (Table 4). This increase is statistically significant ($p = 0.034$). The resource of variety is shown to be a protective factor (beta: –3.8; 95% CI: –0.8 to 0.37), but is not statistically significant. Age reduces the burnout value by 0.6 points per year (95% CI: –0.87 to –0.29), a statistically significant effect ($p < 0.001$). Participation in

Publikation 2

Koch *et al. Journal of Occupational Medicine and Toxicology* (2017) 12:16

Page 5 of 9

Table 2 Resources and stress variables and outcomes at the time of baseline and follow-up (n = 106)

	Baseline				Follow Up				
Resources	x̄	SD	%	n	x̄	SD	%	n	p
Control (scale: 1–5)	3.7	0.9	.	.	3.6	0.9	.	.	0.228
Variety (scale: 1–5)	3.9	0.7	.	.	3.9	0.6	.	.	0.732
Completeness (scale: 1–5)	3.7	0.8	.	.	3.5	0.9	.	.	0.057
Collaboration (scale: 1–5)	3.7	0.7	.	.	3.5	0.8	.	.	0.006*
Information and employee participation (scale: 1–5)	3.8	0.7	.	.	3.7	0.8	.	.	0.120
Stress factors									
Qualitative workload (scale: 1–5)	2.4	0.8	.	.	2.4	0.8	.	.	0.901
Physical stress (scale: 5–20)	14.3	2.8	.	.	14.3	2.8	.	.	0.792
Subjective noise exposure (scale: 13–65)	39.7	10.3	.	.	40.6	10.5	.	.	0.220
ERI ratio score (scale: 0.2–5)	1.2	0.4	.	.	1.3	0.3	.	.	< 0.001**
ERI > 1, proportion (n)	.	.	65.1	69	.	.	87.4	90	< 0.001**
OVC (scale: 6–24)	15.8	3.4	.	.	15.3	3.5	.	.	0.084
Outcomes									
Burnout (scale 0–100)	50.6	19.7	.	.	53.7	20.7	.	.	0.056
Risk of burnout >50,	.	.	53.8	57	.	.	61.3	65	0.096
Neck pain	.	.	32.1	34	.	.	39.4	41	0.286
Shoulder pain	.	.	15.1	16	.	.	19.2	20	0.523
Lower back pain	.	.	39.6	42	.	.	34.6	36	0.523
MS total	.	.	55.7	59	.	.	62.1	64	0.700

x̄: mean, SD: standard deviation, *$p < 0.05$, **$p < 0.001$

the intervention programme has a slightly reductive effect on the target variable (beta: −2.4; 95% CI: −8.66 to 3.78). This effect is not statistically significant. In addition, it can also be observed that the burnout value for employees from child day care centres is 7 points higher than for employees from the two other types of institution (95% CI: 0.56 to 13.51). This increase is statistically significant ($p = 0.034$).

Discussion

In this longitudinal study, statistically significant associations between an increased ERI ratio score and the increase of MS were observed in childcare workers. In these analyses physical stress was included as a confounder variable. With regard to increasing the risk of burnout, ERI was also shown to be a statistically significant factor.

Effort-reward imbalance

We found a high prevalence of ERI among childcare workers (follow-up: 87.4% with ERI ratio > 1; mean ERI ratio: 1.3) in this study, compared to the cross-sectional study from the previous year with a prevalence rate of 65% and a mean ERI ratio of 1.17 [2].

Such unusually high levels of ERI are rare in literature. In an older study investigating childcare workers in 2004, the mean ERI was 0.5 [26]. More recent data assessed in 2012 showed ERI prevalence rates of between 64% and 67% for childcare workers, while for management staff rates of 87% [3, 4]. As was already discussed in the cross-sectional study [2], the increase in ERI over time could potentially be explained by

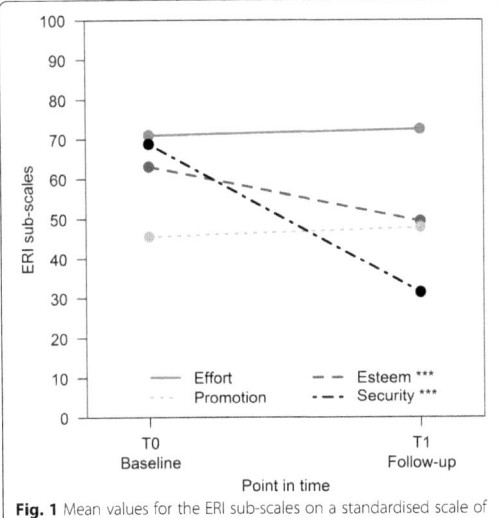

Fig. 1 Mean values for the ERI sub-scales on a standardised scale of 0 to 100 (***$p < 0.001$)

Koch *et al. Journal of Occupational Medicine and Toxicology* (2017) 12:16

Table 3 Results of the multivariate logistic regressions for development of musculoskeletal symptoms (adjusted for age, MS T0)

Outcome at Follow Up:	Lower back 36 (35%)			Shoulder 20 (19%)			Neck 41 (39%)			MS total 64 (62%)		
	OR	95% CI	p	OR	95% CI	p	OR	95% CI	p	OR	95% CI	p
Influencing variables at baseline:												
ERI >1 vs ≤1	4.2*	1.14–15.50	0.031	1.5	0.40–5.58	0.547	4.3*	1.25–15.00	0.021	4.0*	1.20–13.49	0.024
Physical stress high vs low	2.8	0.94–8.10	0.064	1.1	0.33–3.69	0.876	0.9	0.33–2.61	0.891	1.2	0.37–3.87	0.758
Intervention yes vs. no	0.6	0.19–1.86	0.375	2.0	0.63–6.23	0.245	0.9	0.30–2.56	0.804	0.5	0.13–1.63	0.212
OVC 3rd tertile vs 1st + 2nd tertile	.	.	.	0.4	0.09–1.40	0.138	.	.	.	.	.	.
Control high vs low	.	.	.	4.5*	1.15–17.42	0.031	.	.	.	2.0	0.61–6.69	0.254
Physical activity yes vs no	.	.	.	.	.	.	.	.	.	0.3*	0.10–0.98	0.046
Conflicts with parents yes vs no	.	.	.	.	.	.	.	.	.	4.9*	1.55–15.75	0.007
R^2	$R^2 = 0.44$			$R^2 = 0.19$			$R^2 = 0.39$			$R^2 = 0.45$		

*$p < 0.05$

increasing dissatisfaction with working conditions among childcare workers: since 2013, parents in Germany have had a legal right to a childcare place for infants aged 1 to <3, additionally to the existing claim for children aged 3 to 6. In recent years, this has led to larger group sizes, unfavourable staffing conditions and an increase in temporary working contracts. As a result, there was a wave of strikes instigated by childcare workers in Germany in 2015. The questionnaires were returned just a few months after the strikes had taken place. This professional-policy environment is linked with increased awareness of the lack of value accorded to this occupational group in Germany, which is made clear by the drop in the ERI sub-scale *esteem*. The decline in the *job security* sub-scale is also very clear. Paradoxically, almost all staff in the institutions had permanent contracts at the time. The decrease in the two-item *job security* sub-scale was caused in detail by the low scores for the item: "My own job is at risk". Discussion with employee representatives and the management revealed, that at the time of the follow-up the majority of employees were subject to an internal rotation process in their job. This principle meant that, at that time, employees often switched jobs within an institution or between institutions. In this context, answers to this question on the ERI questionnaire were bound to have been biased.

The prevention of ERI by using an ERI model based worksite stress management program, as demonstrated in interventional studies, is feasible and can positively influence psychosocial work environment and mental health [36, 37]. Aiming to reduce overcommitted work-related attitudes, Aust et al. conducted successfully interventions that were performed on individual and organisational levels [36]. With a participative approach Bourbonnais et al. involved employees of a hospital in formulating goals in terms of psychological demands and rewards. After 12 months a reduction of adverse psychological factors was investigated in the experimental group [37].

Musculoskeletal symptoms

We found significant associations between ERI and MS in three out of four body regions in qualified childcare workers: back, neck and combination of back, neck and shoulder (MS total). The association between ERI and lower back pain (OR: 4.2) has been observed in other longitudinal studies investigating employees of a transport company [14], employees in public administration [15] and in other cross-sectional studies investigating employees in healthcare, the wine-growing industry, the police and public transport companies [38–41].

There was a tendency towards association between ERI and the increase of shoulder pain in this study (OR: 1.5)

Table 4 Multivariate linear model for burnout (adjusted for burnout T0)

R^2: 0.53	Regression coefficient	Standardised beta coefficient	95% CI	p
Increase in the ERI ratio score by 10%	1.1*	0.18	0.09–2.14	0.034
Variety (scale 1–5)	−3.8	−0.14	−8.0 – 0.37	0.074
Intervention yes vs no	−2.4	−0.06	−8.66 – 3.78	0.439
Age (per year)	−0.6*	−0.29	−0.87 – −0.29	0.001
Child day care centres yes vs other institutions	7.0*	0.16	0.56–13.51	0.034

*$p < 0.05$
**$p < 0.001$

Publikation 2

Koch *et al. Journal of Occupational Medicine and Toxicology* (2017) 12:16

Page 7 of 9

but not to a statistically significant degree. Lower control (OR: 4.5) was revealed to be a significant influencing factor with regard to shoulder pain. Control as a psychosocial factor derives from the demand-control-support model [42], another stress model that describes the onset of work-related stress.

With regards to neck pain the ERI variable showed a significant effect (OR: 4.3). This effect was also observed in drivers and office workers as well as in cohorts of hospital staff and workers in the wine-growing industry in two longitudinal studies [14, 15] and three cross-sectional studies [38, 39, 43].

For the outcome of total MS, an increased risk was observed for participants with an ERI >1 (OR: 4.0).

Additionally, two other variables seemed to have had an influence on total MS: perceived conflicts with parents (OR: 4.9) and regular physical exercise (OR: 0.3) as a protective factor showed significant associations with the outcome. Childcare workers could be adequately supported with on-the-job training in conflict management to possibly prevent the increase of MS. Conflict management and company-facilitated sports activities for employees would not only directly influence the onset of MS, but would also indirectly affect ERI: childcare workers might perceive this as a kind of esteem for their seniority.

Indications of an interaction between ERI and OVC were not observed in relation to MS. To our knowledge, there is only one cross-sectional study where an interactive effect of this kind was documented with regard to MS in nursing staff [9].

Regarding the biological plausibility there are several explanations for the mechanism of psychosocial factors leading to MS: psychosocial stress might induce increased and prolonged muscle tension [44] and decreased blood supply in extremities [45]. It also blocks anabolic activity which is responsible for the repair of muscle tissue [46]. Another short-term stress response is muscle violation due to increased sensitivity of muscle fibres [44]. Due to these permanent short term responses the risk of chronic MS might increase over time.

Burnout

The prevalence of burnout at the time of the follow-up was higher, at 61.3% (mean: 53.7), than in the cross-sectional study one year before (56.8%, mean: 51.7) [2]. The reference data from the COPSOQ database from 2013 shows a mean burnout score for childcare workers of 48 (Additional file 1, Nuebling). The results of the linear regression showed a significant increase in burnout with an increase in ERI ratio (if the ERI ratio increases by 10%, the burnout risk increases by 1.12 points). In a longitudinal study, Spence et al. [47] also observed a significant association between ERI and

burnout in nurse managers. Other cross-sectional studies have confirmed this association in childcare workers and teaching staff [26, 48, 49]. In contrast to the cross-sectional study [2], however, the association with the ERI model component OVC could not be confirmed in the follow-up. As a personality trait, OVC is a good predictor of burnout and this has been confirmed in a range of studies [27, 50–52]. The analysis also revealed that the burnout value for employees working in child care centres was around seven points higher on average than for employees from school partnership or youth organisations. ERI and burnout prevention measures should therefore be carried out, in particular, among employees working in child care centres.

Limitations

One limitation of the study was the relatively small sample size. This resulted in wide confidence intervals and imprecise evaluations of the estimators. Furthermore, the relatively low follow-up rate resulted in a potential bias in the sample. A non-responder questionnaire was not carried out. On the basis of a dropout analysis, we attempted to identify potential selection effects and to take these into account.

Influential and outcome variables came from the same source – the presence of bias resulting from common methods, such as through social desirability, for example, could therefore not be excluded [53]. The factors of the ERI model only recorded part of the psychosocial situation in the workplace – no other psychosocial factors, such as those used in the job demand-control-support model [42], for example, were used – with the exception of control. Effects of a spill-over of psychosocial factors, but also biomechanical stress from employees' private lives, also could not be excluded since these factors were not recorded as part of the study. Furthermore, part of the sample population (31%) took part in a parallel occupational preventive programme for the reduction of subjective noise exposure [28]. Although the study did not appear to have a statistically significant intervention effect, there were indications that the intervention group showed some benefits in terms of burnout as compared with the reference group. This subgroup was tested in the analyses of MS and burnout, but this characteristic was not shown to have any statistically significant influence. Despite this, it cannot be ruled out that the intervention may have had an effect on the individual level.

Over time, this study shows high and rising rates of burnout and ERI. As mentioned above, we cannot rule out that the professional-policy environment may have resulted in a classification bias of ERI, burnout and MS at

Publikation 2

Koch *et al. Journal of Occupational Medicine and Toxicology* (2017) 12:16

Page 8 of 9

the time that the data was collected. It is highly feasible that the protest movement by childcare workers in Germany at the time that the data was collected had sensitised the study participants and affected their responses.

For the high-risk group identified in the ERI model, those who showed an increased ERI and increased OVC were not shown to have an increased health risk in our study with regard to the outcome variables tested. Taking into account the study limitations, however, childcare workers with an effort-reward imbalance at baseline were shown to have an increased health risk with regard to MS and burnout at follow up.

The small sample size of childcare workers in Hamburg may not be representative for Germany, nevertheless, in comparison to a representative study of German childcare workers [3] there were no differences with respect to age, gender and nationality.

Strengths

The main strength of this study was its longitudinal design. The analyses referred to prevalence rates at time of follow up and controlled for the outcome at baseline. The interpretation of the relation between independent and dependent variable was based on the chronology of time. Another strength, while investigating the relation between psychosocial factors and MS, was the assessment of physical stress and controlling for it in the models. By this approach we controlled a potential confounding effect of physical stress on the association of ERI and MS. Furthermore the assessment of psychosocial factors was performed with a validated instrument which was developed on the basis of a theoretical work stress model. With this approach the development of preventive measures is predetermined by the theory of the ERI model.

Conclusions

As part of an occupational risk assessment, childcare workers were identified as an occupational group with a high ERI prevalence. In this context ERI was identified as a risk factor with regard to burnout and MS as part of a longitudinal approach. Measures should be developed at company level that can help to counter the increase of an effort-reward imbalance. Since monetary changes are hard to carry out at the company level, other measures should be implemented at this level to promote the sense of reward and decrease efforts. These may include the development of a culture that values and recognises its staff, which can be initiated at the management level. There are already empirical indications about the feasibility and success of ERI model based interventions aiming at a positive psychosocial work environment.

Additional file

Additional file 1: Supporting information: Statement Personal Burnout COPSOQ Database. (PDF 97 kb)

Abbreviations
BMI: Body mass index; ERI: Effort-reward imbalance; MS: Musculoskeletal symptoms; OR: Odds ratio; OVC: Overcommitment

Funding
No funding was received.

Availability of data and materials
The datasets generated and/or analysed during the current study are not publicly available due to the fact, that it was not explained in the informed consent form that data would be passed on to other researchers. The data are available from the corresponding author on reasonable request.

Authors' contributions
PK, performed the survey, carried out the statistical analyses and wrote the manuscript. JFK carried out statistical analyses and was critically reading the manuscript. JS read the draft critically and gave substantial comments for the improvement of the first draft. AN revised the manuscript critically for important intellectual content and gave final approval for the version to be published. All authors read and approved the final manuscript.

Ethics approval and consent to participate
Before the study started, every participant gave informed written consent for taking part in the study.
All study documents, including the study protocol, were reviewed and approved by the Hamburg Medical Chamber ethics committee as part of an application process (reference: PV4792).

Consent for publication
Not applicable

Competing interests
PK has no competing interest. JFK has no competing interest. JS has no competing interest. AN has no competing interest.

Author details
[1]Centre of Excellence for Epidemiology and Health Services Research for Healthcare Professionals (CVcare), University Medical Centre Hamburg-Eppendorf, Martinistrasse 52, 20246 Hamburg, Germany. [2]Health Protection Division (FBG), Institution for Statutory Accident Insurance and Prevention in the Health and Welfare Services (BGW), Pappelallee 33, 22089 Hamburg, Germany.

Received: 13 February 2017 Accepted: 20 June 2017
Published online: 26 June 2017

References
1. Siegrist J. Adverse health effects of high-effort/low-reward conditions. J Occup Health Psychol. 1996;1:27–41.
2. Koch P, Stranzinger J, Nienhaus A, Kozak A. Musculoskeletal Symptoms and Risk of Burnout in Child Care Workers - A Cross-Sectional Study. PLoS One. 2015;10:e0140980.
3. Schreyer I, Krause M, Brandl M, Nicko O. AQUA Arbeitsplatz und Qualität in Kitas Ergebnisse einer bundesweiten Befragung. München: Staatsinstitut für Frühpädagogik; 2014.
4. Viernickel S, Voss A, Mauz E, Gerstenberg F, Schumann M. STEGE - Strukturqualität und Erzieher_innengesundheit in Kindertageseinrichtungen. Wissenschaftlicher Abschlussbericht. http://www.gew.de/index.php?eID=dumpFile&t=f&f=20674&token=9d0413d1612a043e64cd74e9e71d51fccefd13ec&download=. Last access 05/22/2017.
5. Siegrist J, Dragano N. Psychosoziale Belastungen und Erkrankungsrisiken im Erwerbsleben. Bundesgesundheitsblatt-Gesundheitsforschung-Gesundheitsschutz. 2008;51(3):305–12.

Publikation 2

Koch *et al. Journal of Occupational Medicine and Toxicology* (2017) 12:16   Page 9 of 9

6. von Kanel R, Bellingrath S, Kudielka BM. Overcommitment but not effort-reward imbalance relates to stress-induced coagulation changes in teachers. Ann Behav Med. 2009;37(1):20–8.
7. Bellingrath S, Rohleder N, Kudielka BM. Healthy working school teachers with high effort–reward-imbalance and overcommitment show increased pro-inflammatory immune activity and a dampened innate immune defence. Brain Behav Immun. 2010;24(8):1332–9.
8. Jolivet A, Caroly S, Ehlinger V, Kelly-Irving M, Delpierre C, Balducci F, et al. Linking hospital workers' organisational work environment to depressive symptoms: A mediating effect of effort-reward imbalance? The ORSOSA study. Soc Sci Med. 2010;71(3):534–40.
9. Weyers S, Peter R, Boggild H, Jeppesen HJ, Siegrist J. Psychosocial work stress is associated with poor self-rated health in Danish nurses: a test of the effort-reward imbalance model. Scand J Caring Sci. 2006; 20:26–34.
10. Buch M, Frieling E. Belastungs- und Beanspruchungsoptimierung in Kindertagesstätten. Kassel: Eigenverlag Universität Kassel, Institut für Arbeitswissenschaft; 2001.
11. Grant KA, Habes DJ, Tepper AL. Work activities and musculoskeletal complaints among preschool workers. Appl Ergon. 1995;26:405–10.
12. Botzet M, Frank H. Arbeit und Gesundheit von Mitarbeiterinnen in Kindertageseinrichtungen. Regionalfallstudie in saarländischen Kindertageseinrichtungen. Landesarbeitsgemeinschaft für Gesundheitsförderung Saarland e.V: Saarbrücken; 1998.
13. Gratz RR, Claffey A. Adult health in childcare: health status, behaviors, and concerns of teachers, directots, and family child care providers. Early Child Res Q. 1996;11:243–67.
14. Rugulies R, Krause N. Effort-reward imbalance and incidence of low back and neck injuries in San Francisco transit operators. Occup Environ Med. 2008;65:525–33.
15. Lapointe J, Dionne CE, Brisson C, Montreuil S. Effort-reward imbalance and video display unit postural risk factors interact in women on the incidence of musculoskeletal symptoms. Work. 2013;44:133–43.
16. Krause N, Burgel B, Rempel D. Effort-reward imbalance and one-year change in neck-shoulder and upper extremity pain among call center computer operators. Scand J Work Environ Health. 2010;36:42–53.
17. Koch P, Schablon A, Latza U, Nienhaus A. Musculoskeletal pain and effort-reward imbalance–a systematic review. BMC Public Health. 2014;14:37.
18. Schaufeli WB, Buunk BP. Burnout. An overview of 25 years of research and theorizing. In: Schabracq MJ, Winnubst JA, Cooper CL, editors. The handbook of work and health psychology. 2nd edn edition. New York: Wiley & Sons; 2003. p. 383–425.
19. Manlove EE. Multiple correlates of burnout in child care workers. Early Child Res Q. 1993;8:499–518.
20. Kushnir T, Milbauer V. Managing stress and burnout at work. A cognitive group intervention. Program for directors of day care centers. Pediatrics. 1994;94:1074–7.
21. Whitebook M, Howes C, Darrah R, Friedman J. Who's minding the child care workers? A look at staff burnout. Child Today. 1980;10:2–6.
22. Bertolino B, Thompson K. The residential youth care worker in action. Binghamton, New York: Hawthorn Press; 1999.
23. Snow K. Aggression: Just part of the job? The psychological impact of aggression on child and youth workers. J Child Youth Care. 1994;9:11–30.
24. Rudow B. Belastungen im Erzieher/innenberuf. Bildung Wissenschaft. 2004;6:6–11.
25. Jungbauer J, Ehlen S. Stress and Burnout Risk in Nursery School Teachers: Results from a Survey. Gesundheitswesen. 2015;77:418–23.
26. Scheuch K, Seibt R. Arbeits- und persönlichkeitsbedingte Beziehungen zu Burnout - eine kritische Betrachtung. In: Richter PG, Rau R, Mühlpfordt S, editors. Arbeit und Gesundheit. Lengerich: Pabst Science Publishers; 2007. p. 42–54.
27. Nübling M, Seidler A, Garthus-Niegel S, Latza U, Wagner M, Hegewald J, et al. The Gutenberg Health Study: measuring psychosocial factors at work and predicting health and work-related outcomes with the ERI and the COPSOQ questionnaire. BMC Public Health. 2013;13:538.
28. Koch P, Stranzinger J, Kersten JF, Nienhaus A. Use of moulded hearing protectors by child care workers - an interventional pilot study. J Occup Med Toxicol. 2016;11:50.
29. Slesina W. FEBA. Fragebogen zur subjektiven Einschätzung der Belastungen am Arbeitsplatz. http://www.rueckenkompass.de/out.php?idart=18. Last access: 05/23/2017.
30. Siegrist J, Starke D, Chandola T, Godin I, Marmot M, Niedhammer I, et al. The measurement of effort-reward imbalance at work: European comparisons. Soc Sci Med. 2004;58:1483–99.
31. Prümper J, Hartmannsgruber K, Frese M. KFZA - Kurzfragebogen zur Arbeitsanalyse. Zeitschrift für Arbeits- und Organisationspsychologie. 1995; 39:125–32.
32. Kuorinka I, Jonsson B, Kilbom A, Vinterberg H, Biering-Sorensen F, Andersson G, et al. Standardised Nordic questionnaires for the analysis of musculoskeletal symptoms. Appl Ergon. 1987;18:233–7.
33. Kristensen TS, Hannerz H, Hogh A, Borg V. The Copenhagen Psychosocial Questionnaire–a tool for the assessment and improvement of the psychosocial work environment. Scand J Work Environ Health. 2005;31:438–49.
34. Hosmer DW, Lemeshow S. Applied logistic regression. New York: Wiley & Sons; 2000.
35. Siegrist J, Li J. Associations of Extrinsic and Intrinsic Components of Work Stress with Health: A Systematic Review of Evidence on the Effort-Reward Imbalance Model. Int J Environ Res Public Health. 2016;13(4):432.
36. Aust B, Peter R, Siegrist J. Stress Management in Bus Drivers: A Pilot Study Based on the Model of Effort–Reward Imbalance. Int J Stress Manag. 1997; 4(4):297–305.
37. Bourbonnais R, Brisson C, Vinet A, Vezina M, Abdous B, Gaudet M. Effectiveness of a participative intervention on psychosocial work factors to prevent mental health problems in a hospital setting. Occup Environ Med. 2006;63(5):335–42.
38. Simon M, Tackenberg P, Nienhaus A, Estryn-Behar M, Conway PM, Hasselhorn HM. Back or neck-pain-related disability of nursing staff in hospitals, nursing homes and home care in seven countries–results from the European NEXT-Study. Int J Nurs Stud. 2008;45:24–34.
39. Bernard C, Courouve L, Bouée S, Adjémian A, Chrétien JC, Niedhammer I. Biomechanical and psychosocial work exposures and musculoskeletal symtoms among vineyard workers. J Occup Health. 2011;53:297–311.
40. von dem Knesebeck O, David K, Siegrist J. Psychosocial stress at work and musculoskeletal pain among police officers in special forces. Gesundheitswesen. 2005;67:674–9.
41. Dragano N, von dem Knesebeck O, Rodel A, Siegrist J. Psychosoziale Arbeitsbelastungen und muskulo-skeletale Beschwerden: Bedeutung für die Prävention. J Public Health. 2003;11:196–207.
42. Karasek RA. Job Demands, Job Decision Latitude, and Mental Strain: Implications for Job Redesign. Adm Sci Q. 1979;24:285–308.
43. Gillen M, Yen IH, Trupin L, Swig L, Rugulies R, Mullen K, et al. The association of socioeconomic status and psychosocial and physical workplace factors with musculoskeletal injury in hospital workers. Am J Ind Med. 2007;50:245–60.
44. Lundberg U, Dohns IE, Melin B, Sandsjö L, Palmerud G, Kadefors R, et al. Psychophysiological stress responses, muscle tension, and neck and shoulder pain among supermarket cashiers. J Occup Health Psychol. 1999;4(3):245.
45. Schleifer LM, Ley R, Spalding TW. A hyperventilation theory of job stress and musculoskeletal disorders. Am J Ind Med. 2002;41(5):420–32.
46. Theorell T, Emdad R, Arnetz B, Weingarten A. Employee Effects of an Educational Program for Managers at an Insurance Company. Psychosom Med. 2001;63:724–33.
47. Spence Laschinger HK, Finegan J. Situational and dispositional predictors of nurse manager burnout: a time-lagged analysis. J Nurs Manag. 2008;16:601–7.
48. Loerbroks A, Meng H, Chen ML, Herr R, Angerer P, Li J. Primary school teachers in China: associations of organizational justice and effort-reward imbalance with burnout and intentions to leave the profession in a cross-sectional sample. Int Arch Occup Environ Health. 2014;87:695–703.
49. Gluschkoff K, Elovainio M, Kinnunen U, Mullola S, Hintsanen M, Keltikangas-Jarvinen L, et al. Work stress, poor recovery and burnout in teachers. Occup Med (Lond). 2016;66:564–70.
50. Lau B. Effort-reward imbalance and overcommitment in employees in a Norwegian municipality: a cross sectional study. J Occup Med Toxicol. 2008;3:9.
51. Wang Y, Ramos A, Wu H, Liu L, Yang X, Wang J, et al. Relationship between occupational stress and burnout among Chinese teachers: a cross-sectional survey in Liaoning. China Int Arch Occup Environ Health. 2015;88:589–97.
52. Chou LP, Li CY, Hu SC. Job stress and burnout in hospital employees: comparisons of different medical professions in a regional hospital in Taiwan. BMJ Open. 2014;4:e004185.
53. Podsakoff PM, MacKenzie SB, Lee JY, Podsakoff NP. Common method biases in behavioral research: a critical review of the literature and recommended remedies. J Appl Psychol. 2003;88:879–903.

Koch *et al. Journal of Occupational Medicine and Toxicology* (2016) 11:50
DOI 10.1186/s12995-016-0138-1

Journal of Occupational
Medicine and Toxicology

RESEARCH   **Open Access**

CrossMark

Use of moulded hearing protectors by child care workers - an interventional pilot study

Peter Koch[1*], Johanna Stranzinger[2], Jan Felix Kersten[1] and Albert Nienhaus[1,2]

Abstract

Background: Employees of a multi-site institution for children and adolescents started to wear moulded hearing protectors (MHPs) during working hours, as they were suffering from a high level of noise exposure. It was agreed with the institutional physician and the German Institution for Statutory Accident Insurance and Prevention in the Health and Welfare Services (BGW) that this presented an opportunity to perform a scientific study to investigate potential beneficial effects on risk of burnout and subjective noise exposure at work when child care workers wear MHPs.

Methods: This was an intervention study which compared the initial values with those after a follow-up of 12 months. All teaching child care workers employed by the multi-site institution were offered the opportunity to take part. Forty-five (45) employees in 16 institutions participated. The subjects were provided with personally adapted MHPs and documented the periods of wear in a diary. At the start and end of the intervention, the subjects had to answer a questionnaire related to subjective noise exposure and burnout risk. In parallel, employees were surveyed who had not taken part in the intervention.

Results: Thirty-three (33) subjects took part in the follow-up after 12 months (follow-up rate 73 %). The median period of wear of MHPs was 34.6 h. During the period of observation, the mean subjective noise exposure increased by 2.7 %, and mean burnout risk by 2.5 scale points (baseline: 55.2, follow-up 57.7). Neither difference was statistically significant. 67 % of the participants reported that they were still capable of fulfilling their teaching duties when wearing the MHPs. In the reference group without the intervention, the increase in burnout risk was 3.9 points, which was even less favourable (baseline: 50.6, follow-up: 54.5).

Conclusions: Within the working environment of the child care workers, wearing MHPs did not reduce subjective noise exposure or burnout risk; satisfaction of the study subjects with wearing MHPs decreased over time. There were however signs that the level of stress increased over time and that this might have been alleviated in the intervention group by wearing MHPs.

Keywords: Moulded hearing protectors, Child care worker, Burnout, Personal hearing protector, Noise exposure

Background

Child care workers in day care centres or other institutions for children and adolescents are continuously exposed to noise from children throughout the working day. Objective measurements have found that the peak sound pressure in these institutions is greater than 85 dB(A) [1–5], which confirms the employees' subjective impression [1, 6, 7]. This noise is mostly caused by the children's voices and their playing [4]. This may be

exacerbated by poor conditions, for example, if the ratio of children to child care workers is high, or if the structure of the building is unsuitable. Studies have shown that staff report fewer health problems when they work in institutions with closed rooms than in those with large half open or open rooms [8]. In this setting, symptoms associated with noise include headache, exhaustion, burnout, stress, voice problems, hearing difficulties and tinnitus [4, 7–12]. In environments with continuous background noise, small children are even at risk of disturbances in speech development [13]. A study with preschool children has shown that children who are exposed to a higher level of noise are more likely to have problems in learning to read [14].

* Correspondence: p.koch@uke.de
[1]Centre of Excellence for Epidemiology and Health Services Research for Healthcare Professionals (CVcare), University Medical Centre Hamburg-Eppendorf, Martinistraße 52, Hamburg 20246, Germany
Full list of author information is available at the end of the article

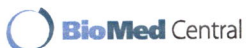

Publikation 3

Koch *et al. Journal of Occupational Medicine and Toxicology* (2016) 11:50

Page 2 of 10

The most usual interventions to reduce noise in child day care centres are technical or organisational. These include, for example, increased noise insulation, the selection of special toys and furniture, using noise warning lights, noise education for children or designating withdrawal rooms for the staff. However, studies on these interventions show that they have little efficacy on subjective noise exposure suffered by employees [11, 15].

In the industrial working environment, the efforts to reduce hearing damage are not only technical or organisational, but may be individualised. In Germany, a personal hearing protector is required if noise exposure exceeds 80 dB(A); this is based on EU Directive 2003/10/EU [16] and was incorporated in the Noise and Vibration Occupational Safety Health Ordinance [17]. In workplaces with technical noise, many employees wear a capsule hearing protector, e.g. soldiers, farmers and industrial workers [18–22]; moulded hearing protectors (MHPs) are often worn by professional musicians. In comparison to capsule hearing protectors, MHPs with adjustable otoplasty filter systems have the advantage that speech is still comprehensible with the hearing protector. For example, in occupational medicine, they are selectively used for teachers and child care workers with hyperacusis. We are unaware of any scientific studies on the use of MHPs in child care workers.

In this context, the following questions were examined in our study:

1a. Does the use of MHPs reduce subjective noise exposure among child care workers?
1b. Does the use of MHPs reduce risk of burnout among child care workers?
2. Do child care workers find the use of MHPs to be comfortable and feasible?
3. What are the acoustics (reverberation time) of critical rooms that were identified by an experienced acoustician and are there associations between acoustic properties of the rooms and subjective noise exposure and risk of burnout respectively?

Methods

As part of stress monitoring for child care workers in a multi-site institution for children and adolescents [7], parallel groups of subjects were recruited for an interventional study on reduction in risk of burnout and subjective noise exposure by MHPs. The participation in the study was offered all 400 child care workers in 26 different facilities (Fig. 1). The multi-site institution bears the responsibility for caring for children in three different types of institutions: 1) day care centres for children aged up to 6 years, 2) school partnerships for school children and 3) facilities to support children and adolescents, e.g. sheltered housing groups. A total of 45

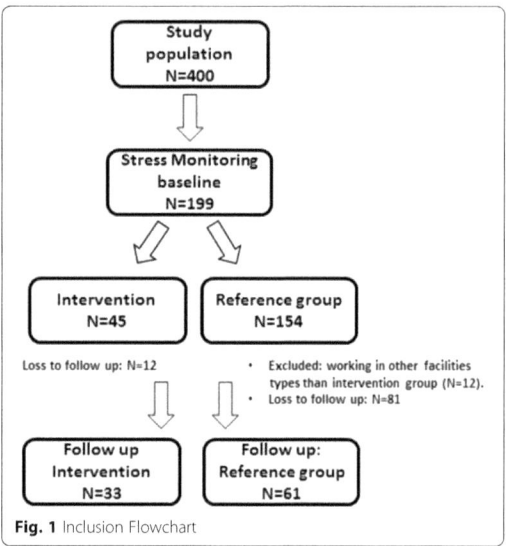

Fig. 1 Inclusion Flowchart

subjects were recruited for the intervention study and also participated in stress monitoring at the same time. The efficacy and practicability of the MHPs were assessed by comparing the initial measurements with those after one year of observation. Post hoc, to examine the results from another perspective, a comparator group was made up of subjects who only took part in stress monitoring. This comparison was carried out so that it would be possible to assess whether the stress potential in the institutions had remained constant or changed over time. As this is not a classical control group, it will be referred to below as the "reference group". 12 subjects working in facilities to support children and adolescents have been excluded from the reference group as in the intervention group no one was working in this type of institution. Overall the reference group comprised 61 subjects. There were no statistically significant differences in demographic characteristics between the intervention and reference group. The inclusion criteria for participation in the intervention were as follows: a) participation in stress monitoring, b) employment in teaching, c) intended employment for at least another year, d) minimum age of 18 years. In order to avoid windfall effects, each subject had to contribute 20 Euros towards their personal hearing protector. The subjects came from 16 different institutions; 11 of these were kindergartens and 5 were school partnerships, in which children from fulltime schools were looked after during teaching breaks.

The pseudoanonymous questionnaire was agreed with the multi-site institution's data protector officer. All study documents including the study protocol were reviewed and approved by the Ethics Committee of the Hamburg

Publikation 3

Koch *et al. Journal of Occupational Medicine and Toxicology* (2016) 11:50

Page 3 of 10

Medical Association (Reference Number: PV4792). Each subject provided a signed declaration of consent.

Intervention

After taking the imprints of the outer ear, the audiologist presented the 45 subjects with a workshop on dealing with MHPs and on the issue of noise. A central recommendation of the workshop was to use the MHPs punctually in situations with high noise exposure (e.g. during lunch). The intervention started in October 2014 (T0) and the subjects were then sent their individually prepared MHPs (Variphone "MEP-2G" Hearing Protector) by post and completed the form on stress monitoring. At the same time, they were given a diary, in which they had to document the times they used the personal hearing protector each day. After five months (T1), the subjects had the opportunity of visiting the audiologist again, in order to modify the fit and the filter strength of their MHPs. At this time, the user satisfaction was recorded with a short questionnaire. After a total of 12 months (T2) follow-up, questionnaires were distributed again on stress monitoring and user satisfaction.

Questionnaire

The questionnaire on stress monitoring collected data on the following factors that could potentially influence the effect of the intervention: three standardized questionnaires components (effort reward imbalance [23], physical stress [24], work-related stress and resources from the Short Questionnaire on Work Analysis (KFZA) [25]). The effort reward imbalance (ERI) questionnaire consists of three dimensions, *effort, reward* and *Overcommitment*. The ERI questionnaire assesses the psychosocial situation of the worker. In studies internal consistencies were satisfactory and varied between 0.70 and 0.91 (Cronbach's alpha) [26, 27]. The KFZA questionnaire comprises different work-related strains and resources. The following scales have been chosen for our questionnaire: *control, variety, entirety, cooperation, qualitative workload, quantitative workload, work disruption and information.* For qualitative workload and work disruption internal consistencies were 0.40 and 0.44 (Cronbachs alpha). For all other scales Cronbachs alpha was between 0.51 and 0.71 [25]. For the questionnaire on physical stress, no study on reliability was available. *Subjective noise exposure* was determined from a cumulative score (range 13–65 points) out of 13 self-developed rating items. Questions such as "There are rooms where I hear particularly poorly" or "This level of noise bothers me" were answered on a 5-point scale, ranging from *strongly agree* to *strongly disagree.* Regarding everyday working life situations for child care workers nine self-developed questions have been added to the questionnaire. To assess situations that might

include a stress potential, questions such as "Breaks and possibilities for recovery are missing" or "There are conflicts with parents" were answered on a 4-point scale ranging from *strongly agree* to *strongly disagree.*

Two outcome variables were examined: burnout risk and subjective noise exposure; the latter may be a factor that influences burnout risk. Burnout risk was assessed on the basis of the subscale *personal burnout* of the Copenhagen Burnout Inventory [28]. In the German version of the Copenhagen Psychosocial Questionnaire (COPSOQ) questionnaire the subscale *personal burnout* shows a Cronbach's alpha of 0.91 [29]. The self-developed questionnaire on user satisfaction collected information on wearing comfort, acoustic perception and the reasonableness of wearing MHPs at work. The answers were rated on the basis of a 5-point rating scale and were then dichotomised due to presentational reasons (yes = absolutely or predominantly true; no = partially correct, predominantly incorrect, absolutely incorrect).

Acoustic measurements

In order to have not only subjective but also objective data on room acoustics, reverberation times were measured in the various institutions during the observation period. The measurements were in the frequency range of 125–4000 Hz and were carried out in rooms with different functions - playrooms, group rooms, classrooms, movement rooms, flights of stairs and restaurants for children. The results were compared with the target values in DIN Norm 18041 on acoustic properties in rooms of small or intermediate size [30]. On the basis of the reverberation times and building properties, an expert in room acoustics performed a final evaluation of the selected rooms. Between 1 and 4 rooms were evaluated for each institution, except one institution of school partnership without any measurement.

Power estimation

During the run-up, it was assumed that about 50 child care workers would be interested in taking part in the study.

On the basis of this number of evaluable cases, it was postulated that the outcome parameter of mean subjective noise exposure would exhibit the necessary normal distribution. With an assumed difference in the means of 2 points before and after the intervention, with a standard deviation of 5 points and an alpha of 5 %, the power of 80 % was calculated.

Statistical analysis

The difference in the means for the comparison before and after the intervention was calculated with the t test for dependent samples, for not normally distributed and dependent data the Wilcoxon signed-rank test was used. Group comparisons were based on the t test for

Publikation 3

Koch et al. Journal of Occupational Medicine and Toxicology (2016) 11:50

Page 4 of 10

independent samples. Analysis of variance (ANOVA) and multivariate linear regression were used to test potential factors for the differences in the means of the outcome variables - subjective noise exposure and burn-out risk (T2-T0), all analyses were performed on the individual level. The following factors were measured at T0 and were considered as factors potentially influencing the outcome variable *subjective noise exposure*: *work-related resources, everyday situations at work, effort reward imbalance, overcommitment, physical stress, weekly working hours, type of institution, physical exercise,* and time of *wearing MHPs*. To characterize the cohort demographic variables like age, gender and BMI were assessed too. For the analysis of the outcome variable *burnout risk*, the additional variable *subjective noise exposure* was investigated as a covariate. Independent variables with a level of significance of $p > 0.2$ in the bivariate analysis were excluded from the analyses. In addition, a drop-out analysis with all variables was performed by logistic regression. If there were statistically significant predictors, these were included as covariates in the linear model. Level of significance was set to two-tailed $p < 0.05$. Statistical analysis was performed with the program SPSS Version 22.

Results

After the follow-up period of 12 months, questionnaires had been received from 33 subjects (follow-up rate: 73 %). Table 1 describes the demographic characteristics of the cohort at time T0. Most subjects were women (91 %). The largest age group consisted of subjects between 40 and 50 years old (38 %). 40 % had a BMI of over 25 and 56 % were regularly engaged in sporting activities. At that point in time, 40 % were working fulltime; most worked in child day care centres.

Figure 2 shows the cumulative wearing time in hours; there were no entries for 6 persons in the diaries. The median of the cumulative wearing time was 34.6 h (range: 0–326). The median cumulative number of days on which the MHPs were worn was 25 days (range 0–174 days).

There were no statistically significant differences between the intervention and reference group with respect to the demographic and all other independent variables e.g. effort reward imbalance. Among the outcome variables, only the difference of the baseline values in subjective noise exposure was statistically significant ($p = 0.004$). Table 2 shows the changes in the outcome variables for the two groups. In the intervention group, mean subjective noise exposure increased from 44.5 to 45.7 points over time (reference group: from 38.1 to 39.7). The difference in subjective noise exposure was greater in the reference group than in the intervention group ($\Delta = 1.6$ vs. 1.2). The difference in the development of subjective noise exposure between the two groups was not statistically significant. In

Table 1 Demographic characteristics of the subjects

Variable	N	Percentage
Gender		
Women	41	91.1 %
Men	4	8.9 %
Age in years		
18 to <30	9	20 %
30 to <40	12	26.7 %
40 to <50	17	37.8 %
50+	7	15.6 %
Nationality		
German	43	95.6 %
Other	2	4.4 %
BMI		
< 25	25	55.6 %
≥ 25	18	40 %
Missing	2	4.4 %
Physical exercise		
Regularly	25	55.6 %
None	20	44.4 %
Weekly working hours		
Fulltime	18	40 %
Part time	27	60 %
Institution		
Child day care centre	36	80 %
School partnership	9	20 %
Support for children and adolescents	0	0 %
Total	45	100 %

the intervention group, the burnout risk increased from 55.2 to 57.7 ($\Delta = 2.5$) points. The increase in the reference group was greater - from 50.6 to 54.5 points ($\Delta = 3.9$). None of the differences between the groups was statistically significant.

Table 3 shows the means of the outcome variables subjective noise exposure and burnout risk for the institutions with or without a recommendation for improvements in room acoustics. For subjective noise exposure at time T0, there was a small difference between the two groups (45.8 vs. 42.2, $\Delta = 3.6$). The difference was slightly greater on follow-up (47.7 vs. 42.8, $\Delta = 4.9$). After 12 months, the difference (Δ T2-T0) for participants from institutions with recommendation was greater than for the other group ($\Delta = 1.9$ vs. 0.7) but statistically not significant. The differences in burnout risk were greater: at time point T0 (59.2 vs. 48.3), the difference was 10.9 and, at time point T2 (60.8 vs. 52.1), the difference was 8.7 points on the burnout scale. At time point T2 the differences in burnout risk (Δ T2-T0) for

Publikation 3

Koch *et al. Journal of Occupational Medicine and Toxicology* (2016) 11:50

Page 5 of 10

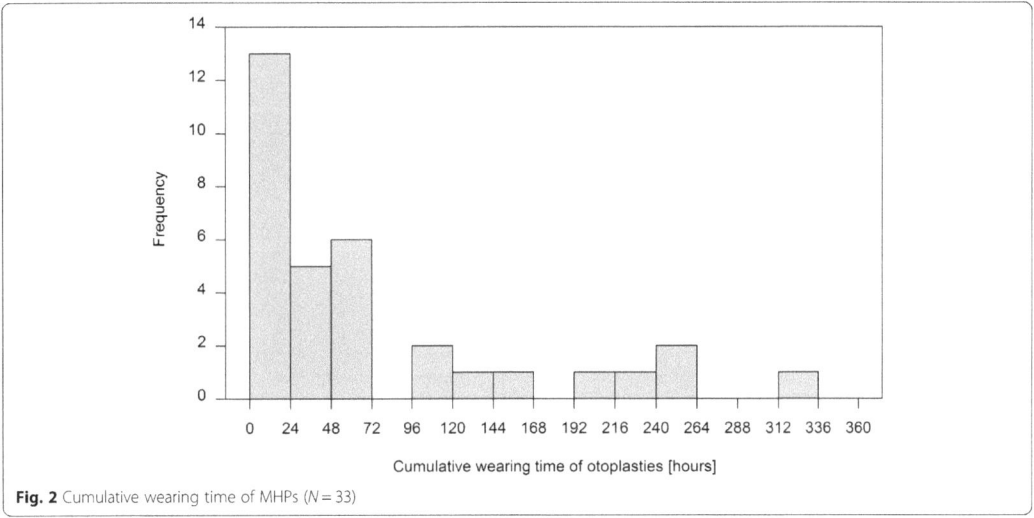

Fig. 2 Cumulative wearing time of MHPs (*N* = 33)

workers from institutions without a recommendation was more than double high than for the comparison group (Δ = 3.8 vs. 1.6) However, none of these differences was statistically significant.

Multivariate analysis demonstrated that the feature *Breaks and possibilities for recovery are missing* had a significant effect on subjective noise exposure (B = 5.7, *p* = 0.013) (Table 4). According to this, the effect on subjective noise exposure for this subgroup became even less favourable over time. All other potential factors exhibited no significant effects and were therefore excluded from the model. No statistically significant effects on burnout were identified.

Figure 3 shows the information on the satisfaction of the study subjects with wearing MHPs at just over the half of the observation period (T1) and at the end of the period (T2). Satisfaction tended to decrease over time. For example, the fraction of those who found it unpleasant to wear hearing protection in the presence of parents rose from 18 to 35 %. The fraction of those who thought

it was reasonable to wear MHPs sank from 69 to 47 %. The fraction of those who experienced relaxation after work remained constant over time (48 %). The fraction of subjects who missed information slightly improved over time - from 27 to 23 %. Almost three quarter of study subjects (72 %) thought that they could fulfil their teaching duties at time point T1. At time point T2 this value decreased to 67 %. None of these changes over time in the dichotomous variables was statistically significant.

Table 5 describes the distribution of study subjects over the 16 different institutions at T0 and T2. The number of subjects at T0 was between one and seven employees per institution. At time point T2, there was no longer any subject from two of the institutions. The number per institution varied between 1 and 5 persons.

Reverberation times were measured between one and a maximum of four rooms in the different institutions (Table 5). No improvements in the room acoustics were evaluated in 6 institutions, as indicated by the reverberation time measurements and other room characteristics.

Table 2 Description of the outcome variables in the intervention and reference groups

	Intervention group (*N* = 33)*			Reference group (*N* = 61)*		
	T0	T2	*p*	T0	T2	*p*
Subjective Noise Exposure	44.5 (8.8)	45.7 (7.9)	0.30	38.1 (10.3)	39.7 (10.5)	0.08
Δ Subjective Noise Exposure T2-T0	1.2 (7.4)		NA	1.6 (6.8)		0.80
Burnout Risk Scale	55.2 (19.4)	57.7 (17.7)	0.40	50.6 (19.7)	54.5 (22.1)	0.05
Δ Burnout Risk Scale T2-T0	2.5 (18.3)		NA	3.9 (15.3)		0.70
Burnout Risk Scale ≥ 50	66.7 %	72.7 %	0.62	54.1 %	62.3 %	0.22

*given values are means (standard deviations), rates and *p*-values

Koch *et al. Journal of Occupational Medicine and Toxicology* (2016) 11:50

Table 3 Outcome variables for subjects in institutions with or without a recommendation for improvement in room acoustics

| | Acoustic improvements recommended? Yes ($N = 20$), No ($N = 12$) | | | | | |
| | Subjective Noise Exposure* | | | Burnout Risk Scale* | | |
	Yes	No	p	Yes	No	p
T0	45.8 (9.3)	42.2 (8.2)	0.26	59.2 (19.9)	48.3 (19.8)	0.13
T2	47.7 (7.2)	42.8 (8.8)	0.12	60.8 (19.6)	52.1 (14.1)	0.15
Δ T2-T0	1.9 (8.2)	0.7 (7.6)	0.67	1.6 (20.7)	3.8 (15.4)	0.75

*given values are means (standard deviations) and p-values

For the other institutions, improvements in room acoustics were recommended for at least one room. In one institution, no measurement could be performed for organisational reasons. The target values for reverberation times depend on the functions and sizes of the rooms; these values were exceeded in 29/39 measurements (74 %).

Discussion

When child care workers used MHPs in the present setting, their subjective noise exposure and risk of burnout was not reduced over the period of observation.

It was also observed that most of the subjects did not consider it to be very reasonable to wear MHPs and that this reduced their ability to fulfil their teaching duties over time.

As regards the room acoustics, improvements in room acoustics were recommended for more than half of the institutions on the basis of the measured reverberation times and the structural properties of the rooms.

Limitations

This study is a scientific investigation of the effect of MHPs. On the other hand, it is also a preventive measure in occupational medicine, which is intended to be available to all employees. In contrast to a classical RCT, this study was performed without a control group or randomisation and without monitoring of other conditions. As a post-hoc analysis the reference group was included to show to what extent the study was performed under changing overall conditions. As the burnout risk was even greater in the reference group, it is clear that there were uncontrolled factors that influenced these outcome variables in both groups. As the threshold for inclusion was low, it can also be assumed that the group was relatively heterogeneous. At the start of the study, the subjects were not subjected to audiometric controls with respect to, for example, hardness of hearing, tinnitus or ear noises, so

that the status of their hearing is unknown. Thus, it remains possible that their hearing was heterogeneous. This has the advantage that an occupational preventive measure should be open to as many employees as possible.

A failure of unknown reason in the implementation of the intervention conclusively led to little cumulative wearing time. Consequently it was statistically unlikely to detect any potential dose–response relationship between the wearing time and outcome variables. Qualitative interviews, that could have shed light upon the reasons for the failed implementation of the intervention, were not performed in this pilot study. Because of the size of the sample and the follow-up rate of 73 %, it was hardly possible to demonstrate statistically significant effects; the expected power of 0.80 was not reached in this study, apart from the unforeseen development of the outcome variables. This also applied to the drop-out analysis. This did not allow any conclusion as to whether there was no selection bias, or whether the low number of participants prevented the demonstration of statistically significant variables. Moreover, the non-responders survey (3 of 12 questionnaires returned) did not permit any reliable conclusion about the reasons for non-participation either.

Measurements of sound pressure would have provided an objective estimate of noise exposure, and there are already reference values from German kindergartens. These measurements - including audiometry - had originally been planned for the start of the study. However, they were postponed for organisational reasons and would finally have had to be carried out a long time after the end of the observational period. We therefore eventually decided to dispense with these measurements.

Intervention

The entry of the wearing times in the diary is intended to be a sort of quality assurance for the intervention. For 6 persons (18 %), there were no entries in the diaries for

Table 4 Results of multivariate linear regression ($N = 32$), adjusted for subjective noise exposure at time point T0

| Dependent variable: Difference in subjective noise exposure T2-T0 | | | |
Factor	Effect	95 % CI	p
Breaks and possibilities for recovery are missing (1 = yes, 0 no)	5.7	1.29–10.13	0.013
	$R^2 = 0.42$		

Koch *et al. Journal of Occupational Medicine and Toxicology* (2016) 11:50

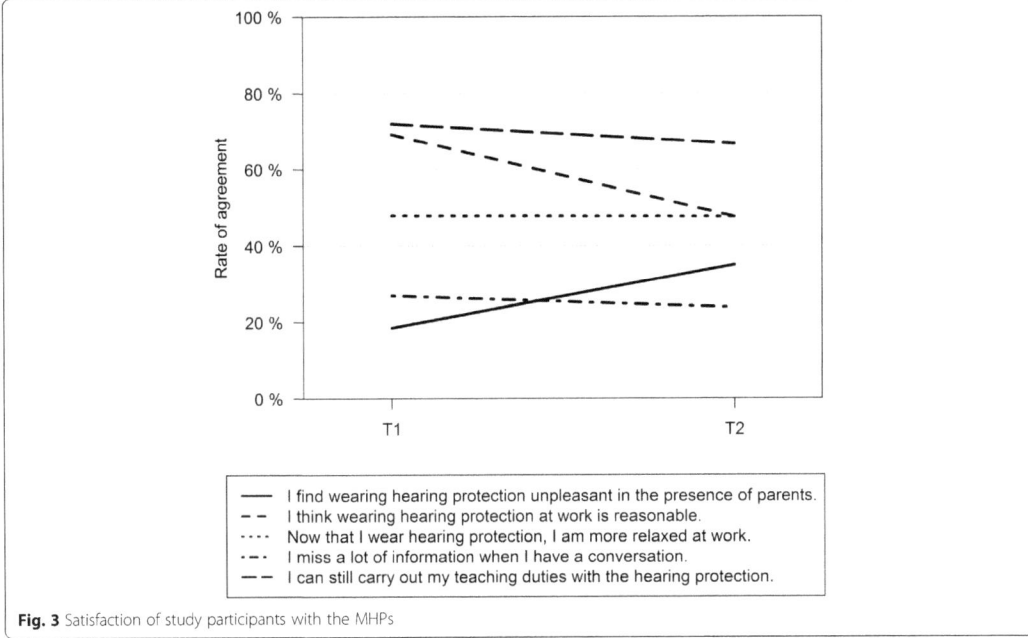

Fig. 3 Satisfaction of study participants with the MHPs

Table 5 Overview of room acoustic measurements

Institutions		Participants		Mean reverberation time in seconds (T0): **(actual)** (target)	Room acoustic improvements recommended by the room acoustics expert
		T0 (N)	T2 (N)		
Child day care centres	C₁	2	2	**0.48** (0.50)	No
	C₂	3	1	**0.46** (0.40), **0.47** (0.40), **0.73** (0.50)	Yes
	C₃	3	3	**0.60** (0.50), **0.45** (0.40), **0.60** (0.40)	No
	C₄	1	0	**0.48** (0.50), **0.60** (0.45), **0.50** (0.40)	No
	C₅	3	2	**0.38** (0.45)	No
	C₆	3	2	**0.48** (0.40), **0.56** (0.50)	Yes
	C₇	3	3	**0.35** (0.40), **0.44** (0.50)	Yes
	C₈	5	4	**0.64** (0.55), **0.49** (0.40), **0.37** (0.40), **0.58** (0.50)	Yes
	C₉	7	5	**0.70** (0.55), **0.54** (0.50), **0.61** (0.50)	Yes
	C₁₀	2	1	**0.53** (0.40), **0.45** (0.40), **0.89** (0.50)	Yes
	C₁₁	4	4	**0.42** (0.50)	No
School partnerships	S₁	1	1	**0.57** (0.55), **0.66** (0.55)	No
	S₂	3	2	**0.47** (0.50), **0.60** (0.50), **0.69** (0.50), **0.73** (0.80)	Yes
	S₃	2	0	**0.85** (0.65), **0.88** (0.65), **0.50** (0.50)	Yes
	S₄	2	2	**0.64** (0.60), **0.82** (0.60), **0.57** (0.50), **0.97** (0.70)	Yes
	S₅	1	1	No measurements	No information

Bold: actual, not bold: target

Koch et al. Journal of Occupational Medicine and Toxicology (2016) 11:50

the wearing times, i.e. it was not known whether these persons had actually worn the MHPs. In accordance with the *intention to treat* principle, these persons were included in the analysis. With the median cumulative wearing time of 34.6 h over 12 months and full employment (224 working days in 2015), this corresponds to a mean daily wearing time of maximally 9 min for half of the participants. As there are no other studies on this type of intervention, there are no reference values and it is difficult to assess whether this is an effective period of time with respect to noise exposure. In the initial workshop, it was emphasised that the participants should wear MHPs at times of peak noise. If time dependent measurements of sound pressure had been performed in the different institutions over the shifts, it might have been possible to relate these to the wearing times. On the other hand, if you consider the statements on satisfaction with MHPs (teaching duties, reasonableness, relaxation effect etc.), it seems more likely that in a substantial number of cases the MHPs were not worn much, because they were disturbing at work.

Comparison with the reference group makes it clear that, at baseline, the intervention group exhibited higher values for both noise exposure and burnout. Especially the difference in subjective noise exposure indicates self-selection of the intervention group. In both groups, burnout risk increased over time. The mean burnout risk and the prevalence in the intervention group (T2: 57.7 and 72.7 %, respectively) appear to be comparatively high. The 2013 COPSOQ database gives a mean reference value of 48 for German child care workers (data in Supporting Information); Buch and Frieling give a burnout prevalence of 30 % [1]. The increase in the burnout risk was smaller in the intervention group, which might indicate that the intervention had a favourable alleviating effect. No factors which might have influenced the intervention effect could be identified in the multivariate analyses. In contrast, it was observed that changes in noise exposure over time were less favourable for subjects who stated in the questionnaire that breaks and possibilities for recovery were missing; thus, the increase in the mean noise exposure values was 5.7 points greater for these persons.

The room acoustic evaluation, including measurements of reverberation time, showed that improvements were possible in 9 of 15 institutions. In some cases, the reverberation times were too high, but in other cases the room acoustics could be improved even though the reverberation times were moderate. Possible problems include wrongly mounted shock absorber elements, missing impact sound insulation, metal doors or too many window surfaces. These assessments make it clear that room acoustics may be suboptimal even when the reverberation times are moderate in accordance with the DIN standard. It was striking - albeit not statistically significant - that employees from institutions where the room acoustics could be improved exhibited higher values of the outcome variables - particularly burnout risk - at both time points. Specific improvements, particularly in these institutions, would therefore benefit the group of employees under the greatest stress. Studies have shown that improvements in room acoustics in schools can reduce reverberation times and, in some cases, also subjective noise exposure [8, 11, 15]. The use of special toy containers can also bring a major reduction in the level of sound pressure [31]. Aside from structural changes, noise exposure can also be reduced at the organisational level. This includes the use of recovery rooms, noise warning lights, light regulation, teaching that increases sensitivity to noise and speech training for child care workers. However, Sjödin et al. have shown that organisational measures are less effective than room acoustic measures, as they require more work [11].

In summary, this study was based on an idea that was initiated by stressed employees and which was implemented as a behavioural preventive measure with scientific support. Due to this frame several characteristics like lack of randomization and control, use of post-hoc reference group, missing compliance in the intervention group and underpowered conditions limit the validity in this study. Further studies should be also designed in a mixed method approach with additional qualitative research. Overall the results suggest that, in this specific setting, wearing MHPs is not an appropriate occupational measure and therefore could not be effectively implemented. In this context it seems that prevention by technical engineering might be more important than the use of personal protective equipment. Qualitative interviews would have been able to identify the reasons for the lack of compliance here more precisely. In contrast to employees in industry, child care workers are exposed to informative noise that has to be heard and which accordingly includes a high level of potential stress. Perhaps the employees' feelings of responsibility to the children prevented them from wearing the MHPs regularly.

The structural causes of the noise exposure and possibly also burnout risk in this group are presumably inadequate numbers of employees, excessively large groups and, especially, too few trained child care workers [7]. These issues have long been discussed by politicians with expertise in employment and could only be modified at another level. In general, the motivation for this study was typical of the overall conditions for child care workers in Germany, with unfavourable ratios of children to child care workers and lack of expert staff.

Publikation 3

Koch *et al. Journal of Occupational Medicine and Toxicology* (2016) 11:50

Page 9 of 10

Conclusion

The use of MHPs by child care workers in child day care centres is not an appropriate measure to prevent noise exposure if it is widely employed. For groups of employees with specific problems such as hyperacusis after acute hearing loss further studies are needed. Within the institutions, a careful analysis should be performed of the room acoustics, followed by modification as necessary. In addition, organisational measures e.g. noise education for children should be implemented that have a favourable effect on the initiation and development of noise and its effects on health.

Abbreviations
BGW: German Social Accident Insurance Institution for the Health and Welfare Services; BMI: Body mass index; COPSOQ: Copenhagen Psychosocial Questionnaire; dB: Decibel; ERI: Effort reward imbalance; KFZA: Short Questionnaire on Work Analysis; MHPs: Moulded hearing protectors

Acknowledgements
We thank Dr. Matthias Nübling for assistance with unpublished data of the Copenhagen Psychosocial Questionnaire (COPSOQ) database.

Funding
The study was funded by the German Institution for Statutory Accident Insurance and Prevention in the Health and Welfare Services (BGW).

Availability of data and materials
As we did not ask for sharing the data with others in the informed consent form, we are obliged to keep the data protected.

Authors' contributions
PK, performed the survey, carried out the statistical analyses and wrote the manuscript. JS read the draft critically and gave substantial comments for the improvement of the first draft. JFK supported the statistical analysis and supported the writing process. AN revised the manuscript critically for important intellectual content and gave final approval for the version to be published. All authors read and approved the final manuscript.

Competing interests
The authors declare that they have no competing interests.

Consent for publication
Not applicable.

Ethics approval and consent to participate
We confirm that the study has been performed in accordance with the Declaration of Helsinki and has been approved by the Ethics Committee of Hamburg Medical Association (Reference Number: PV4792). The pseudoanonymous questionnaire was agreed with the multi-site institution's data protector officer and each subject provided a signed declaration of consent.

Author details
[1]Centre of Excellence for Epidemiology and Health Services Research for Healthcare Professionals (CVcare), University Medical Centre Hamburg-Eppendorf, Martinistraße 52, Hamburg 20246, Germany. [2]Health Protection Division (FBG), Institution for Statutory Accident Insurance and Prevention in the Health and Welfare Services (BGW), Pappelallee 33, Hamburg 22089, Germany.

Received: 22 June 2016 Accepted: 2 November 2016
Published online: 08 November 2016

References
1. Buch M, Frieling E. Belastungs- und Beanspruchungsoptimierung in Kindertagesstätten. Kassel: Eigenverlag Universität Kassel, Institut für Arbeitswissenschaft; 2001.
2. Eysel-Gosepath K, Pape HG, Erren T, Thinschmidt M, Lehmacher W, Piekarski C. Sound levels in nursery schools. HNO. 2010;58:1013–20.
3. Paulsen R. Noise Exposure in Kindergartens. In CFA/DAGA'04 30 Jahrestagung für Akustik - Europäische Akustik-Ausstellung Akustik DGf ed., vol. I. pp. 573–574. Straßburg; 2004:573–574.
4. Sjodin F, Kjellberg A, Knutsson A, Landstrom U, Lindberg L. Noise and stress effects on preschool personnel. Noise Health. 2012;14:166–78.
5. Neitzel RL, Svensson EB, Sayler SK, Ann-Christin J. A comparison of occupational and nonoccupational noise exposures in Sweden. Noise Health. 2014;16:270–8.
6. Losch D. Lärm als Stressor in der Kindertagesstätte. Zentralblatt für Arbeitsmedizin, Arbeitsschutz und Ergonomie. 2016;66:20–8.
7. Koch P, Stranzinger J, Nienhaus A, Kozak A. Musculoskeletal Symptoms and Risk of Burnout in Child Care Workers - A Cross-Sectional Study. PLoS One. 2015;10:e0140980.
8. Truchnon-Gagnon C, Hetu R. Noise in Day-care centers for children. Noise Control Eng J. 1988;30:57–64.
9. Jungbauer J, Ehlen S. Stress and burnout risk in nursery school teachers: results from a survey. Gesundheitswesen. 2015;77:418–23.
10. Sjodin F, Kjellberg A, Knutsson A, Landstrom U, Lindberg L. Noise exposure and auditory effects on preschool personnel. Noise Health. 2012;14:72–82.
11. Sjodin F, Kjellberg A, Knutsson A, Landstrom U, Lindberg L. Measures against preschool noise and its adverse effects on the personnel: an intervention study. Int Arch Occup Environ Health. 2014;87:95–110.
12. Sodersten M, Granqvist S, Hammarberg B, Szabo A. Vocal behavior and vocal loading factors for preschool teachers at work studied with binaural DAT recordings. J Voice. 2002;16:356–71.
13. Niemitalo-Haapola E, Haapala S, Jansson-Verkasalo E, Kujala T. Background Noise Degrades Central Auditory Processing in Toddlers. Ear Hear. 2015;36:e342–51.
14. Maxwell LE, Evans GW. The effects of noise on preschool Chidren's Pre-readiing skills. Journal of Environmental Psychology. 2000;20:91–7.
15. Gerhardsson L, Nilsson E. Noise disturbances in daycare centers before and after acoustical treatment. J Environ Health. 2013;75:36–40.
16. European Union. Richtlinie 2003/10/EG des europäischen Parlaments und des Rates vom 6. Februar 2003 über Mindestvorschriften zum Schutz von Sicherheit und Gesundheit der Arbeitnehmer vor der Gefährdung durch physikalische Einwirkungen (Lärm). 2003. http://eur-lex.europa.eu/legal-content/DE/TXT/PDF/?uri=CELEX:32003L0010&rid=3 Accessed 20 Jun 2016.
17. The Federal Ministry of Justice, Germany. Verordnung zum Schutz der Beschäftigten vor Gefährdungen durch Lärm und Vibrationen. http://www.gesetze-im-internet.de/l_rmvibrationsarbschv/. Accessed 20 Jun 2016.
18. Berg RL, Pickett W, Fitz-Randolph M, Broste SK, Knobloch MJ, Wood DJ, Kirkhorn SR, Linneman JG, Marlenga B. Hearing conservation program for agricultural students: short-term outcomes from a cluster-randomized trial with planned long-term follow-up. Prev Med. 2009;49:546–52.
19. Brink LL, Talbott EO, Burks JA, Palmer CV. Changes over time in audiometric thresholds in a group of automobile stamping and assembly workers with a hearing conservation program. AIHA J. 2002;63:482–7.
20. Erlandsson B, Hakanson H, Ivarsson A, Nilsson P. The difference in protection efficiency between earplugs and earmuffs. An investigation performed at a workplace. Scand Audiol. 1980;9:215–21.
21. Heyer N, Morata TC, Pinkerton LE, Brueck SE, Stancescu D, Panaccio MP, Kim H, Sinclair JS, Waters MA, Estill CF, Franks JR. Use of historical data and a novel metric in the evaluation of the effectiveness of hearing conservation program components. Occup Environ Med. 2011;68:510–7.
22. Verbeek JH, Kateman E, Morata TC, Dreschler WA, Mischke C. Interventions to prevent occupational noise-induced hearing loss: a Cochrane systematic review. Int J Audiol. 2014;53 Suppl 2:S84–96.
23. Siegrist J. Adverse health effects of high-effort/low-reward conditions. J Occup Health Psychol. 1996;1:27–41.
24. Slesina W. FEBA: Fragebogen zur subjektiven Einschätzung der Belastungen am Arbeitsplatz. 2009 http://www.rueckenkompass.de/download_files/doc/Fragen-Slesina.pdf Accessed 20 Jun 2016.
25. Prümper J, Hartmannsgruber K, Frese M. KFZA - Kurzfragebogen zur Arbeitsanalyse. Zeitschrift für Arbeits- und Organisationspsychologie. 1995;39:125–32.

Publikation 3

Koch *et al. Journal of Occupational Medicine and Toxicology* (2016) 11:50

Page 10 of 10

26. Niedhammer I, Siegrist J, Landre MF, Goldberg M, Leclerc A. Psychometric properties of the French version of the Effort-Reward Imbalance model. Rev Epidemiol Sante Publique. 2000;48:419–37.
27. Tsutsumi A, Ishitake T, Peter R, Siegrist J, Matoba T. The Japanese version of the effort-reward imbalance questionnaire: a study in dental technicians. Work & Stress. 2001;15:86–96.
28. Kristensen TS, Hannerz H, Hogh A, Borg V. The Copenhagen psychosocial questionnaire–a tool for the assessment and improvement of the psychosocial work environment. Scand J Work Environ Health. 2005;31:438–49.
29. Nübling M, Stößel U, Hasselhorn H-M, Michaelis M, Hofmann F. Measuring psychological stress and strain at work: Evaluation of the COPSOQ Questionnaire in Germany. GMS Psycho-Social-Medicine. 2006;3:1–14.
30. German Institute for Standardization. DIN 18041:2015–02 Hörsamkeit in Räumen- Vorgaben und Hinweise für die Planung. Beuth; 2015.
31. Scharf T, Groneberg DA. Lärm in deutschen Kindertageseinrichtungen: Eine Pilotstudie mit praktischer Handlungsanweisung zu lärmreduzierenden Maßnahmen. In: RiRe- Risiken und Ressourcen in Gesundheitsdienst und Wohlfahrtspflege. Volume 2. Edited by Nienhaus. Landsberg am Lech: Ecomed Medizin; 2015 p. 75–82

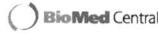

3 Literaturverzeichnis

ArbSchG, *Arbeitsschutzgesetz vom 7. August 1996 (BGBI. I S. 1246), das zuletzt durch Artikel 427 der Verordnung vom 31. August 2015 (BGBI. I S. 1474) geändert worden ist.*

Aust, B., R. Peter and J. Siegrist (1997). *"Stress Management in Bus Drivers: A Pilot Study Based on the Model of Effort–Reward Imbalance". International Journal of Stress Management 4(4): 297-305.*

BAUA, Bundesanstalt für Arbeitsschutz und Arbeitsmedizin (2016). *Sicherheit und Gesundheit bei der Arbeit 2015- Unfallverhütungsbericht Arbeit. Dortmund.*

Berg, R. L., W. Pickett, M. Fitz-Randolph, S. K. Broste, M. J. Knobloch, D. J. Wood, S. R. Kirkhorn, J. G. Linneman and B. Marlenga (2009). *"Hearing conservation program for agricultural students: short-term outcomes from a cluster-randomized trial with planned long-term follow-up".Prev Med 49(6): 546-552.*

Berger, J., D. Niemann, H. Nolting, G. Schiffhorst, H. Genz and M. Kordt (2002). *„Arbeitsbedingungen und Stress bei Erzieher/innen. Ergebnisse des BGW–DAK Stress-Monitorings". IGES Institut für Gesundheits-und Sozialforschung. Berlin.*

Bernard, C., L. Courouve, S. Bouée, A. Adjémian, J. C. Chrétien and I. Niedhammer (2011). *"Biomechanical and psychosocial work exposures and musculoskeletal symtoms among vineyard workers". Journal of Occupational Health 53(5): 297-311.*

Bock-Famulla, K., J., E. Strunz, A. Löhle (2017). *Länderreport Frühkindliche Bildungssysteme 2017, Verlag Bertelsmann Stiftung Gütersloh.*

Bourbonnais, R., C. Brisson and M. Vézina (2011). *"Long-term effects of an intervention on psychosocial work factors among healthcare professionals in a hospital setting". Occupational and Environmental Medicine 68(7): 479-486.*

Bourbonnais, R., C. Brisson, A. Vinet, M. Vezina, B. Abdous and M. Gaudet (2006). *"Effectiveness of a participative intervention on psychosocial work factors to prevent mental health problems in a hospital setting". Occup Environ Med 63(5): 335-342.*

Bright, K. and K. Calabro (1999). *"Child care workers and workplace hazards in the United States: Overview of research and implications for occupational health professionals". Occupational medicine 49(7): 427-437.*

Brink, L. L., E. O. Talbott, J. A. Burks and C. V. Palmer (2002). *"Changes over time in audiometric thresholds in a group of automobile stamping and assembly workers with a hearing conservation program". AIHA J (Fairfax, Va) 63(4): 482-487.*

Buch, M. and E. Frieling (2001). *Belastungs- und Beanspruchungsoptimierung in Kindertagestätten. Kassel, Eigenverlag Universität Kassel, Institut für Arbeitswissenschaft.*

Chou, L. P., C. Y. Li and S. C. Hu (2014). *"Job stress and burnout in hospital employees: comparisons of different medical professions in a regional hospital in Taiwan". BMJ Open 4(2): e004185.*

Cryer, D., W. Tietze, M. Burchinal, T. Leal and J. Palacios (1999). *"Predicting process quality from structural quality in preschool programs: A cross-country comparison". Early Childhood Research Quarterly 14(3): 339-361.*

DIN 18041:2015-02 (2015). *"Hörsamkeit in Räumen – Vorgaben und Hinweise für die Planung". Beuth Verlag. Berlin.*

Dragano, N., O. von dem Knesebeck, A. Rodel and J. Siegrist (2003). *"Psychosoziale Arbeitsbelastungen und muskulo-skeletale Beschwerden: Bedeutung für die Prävention." Journal of Public Health 11(3): 196-207.*

EU (2003). „*Richtlinie 2003/10/EG des Europäischen Parlaments und des Rates vom 6. Februar 2003 über Mindestvorschriften zum Schutz von Sicherheit und Gesundheit der Arbeitnehmer vor der Gefährdung durch physikalische Einwirkungen (Lärm)".* http://eur-lex.europa.eu/legal-content/ DE/TXT/PDF/?uri=CELEX:32003L0010&rid=3 (Stand 20.11.2017).

Erlandsson, B., H. Hakanson, A. Ivarsson and P. Nilsson (1980). *"The difference in protection efficiency between earplugs and earmuffs. An investigation performed at a workplace".* Scand Audiol 9(4): 215-221.

Eysel-Gosepath, K., H. G. Pape, T. Erren, M. Thinschmidt, W. Lehmacher and C. Piekarski (2010). *„Sound levels in nursery schools".* HNO 58(10): 1013-1020.

Fuchs-Rechlin, K. (2007). „*Wie geht's im Job? KiTa-Studie der GEW".* Gewerkschaft Erziehung und Wissenschaft-Hauptvorstand, Organisationsbereich Jugendhilfe und Sozialarbeit/Universität Dortmund, Arbeitsstelle Kinder-und Jugendhilfestatistik (AKJStat).

Fuchs, T. and F. Trischler (2008). „*Arbeitsqualität aus Sicht von Erzieherinnen und Erziehern".* Ergebnisse aus der Erhebung zum DGB-Index Gute Arbeit. http://archiv.verdi-gute-arbeit.de/ upload/m4947cc45d3d5f_verweis1.pdf (Stand 20.11.2017).

Gerhardsson, L. and E. Nilsson (2013). *"Noise disturbances in daycare centers before and after acoustical treatment".* J Environ Health 75(7): 36-40.

Gilbert-Ouimet, M., C. Brisson, M. Vezina, L. Trudel, R. Bourbonnais, B. Masse, G. Baril-Gingras and C. E. Dionne (2011). *"Intervention study on psychosocial work factors and mental health and musculoskeletal outcomes".* Healthc Pap 11 Spec No: 47-66.

Gillen, M., I. H. Yen, L. Trupin, L. Swig, R. Rugulies, K. Mullen, A. Font, D. Burian, G. Ryan, I. Janowitz, P. A. Quinlan, J. Frank and P. Blanc (2007). *"The association of socioeconomic status and psychosocial and physical workplace factors with musculoskeletal injury in hospital workers".* Am J Ind Med 50(4): 245-260.

Gluschkoff, K., M. Elovainio, U. Kinnunen, S. Mullola, M. Hintsanen, L. Keltikangas-Jarvinen and T. Hintsa (2016). *"Work stress, poor recovery and burnout in teachers".* Occup Med (Lond) 66(7): 564-570.

Goelman, H. and H. Guo (1998). *"What we know and what we don't know about burnout among early childhood care providers".* Child and Youth Care Forum 27(3).

Gordis, L. (2001). *Fall-Kontroll-Studien und Querschnittsstudien. Epidemiologie.* Marburg, Verlag im Kilian.

Hall, A. and I. Leppelmeier (2015). „*Erzieherinnen und Erzieher in der Erwerbstätigkeit – Ihre Arbeitsbedingungen, Arbeitsbelastungen und die Folgen".* Bundesinstitut für Berufsbildung. Wissenschaftliches Diskussionspapier 161.

Heyer, N., T. C. Morata, L. E. Pinkerton, S. E. Brueck, D. Stancescu, M. P. Panaccio, H. Kim, J. S. Sinclair, M. A. Waters, C. F. Estill and J. R. Franks (2011). *"Use of historical data and a novel metric in the evaluation of the effectiveness of hearing conservation program components".* Occup Environ Med 68(7): 510-517.

Hinding, B., S. Akca and M. Kastner (2012). „*Wertschätzung als Prädiktor für die Leistungsfähigkeit und Gesundheit des Pegepersonals im Krankenhaus".* Plexus, Supplement 20.

Hoogendoorn, W. E., M. N. van Poppel, P. M. Bongers, B. W. Koes and L. M. Bouter (2000). *"Systematic review of psychosocial factors at work and private life as risk factors for back pain".* Spine 25(16): 2114-2125.

Hosmer, D. W. and S. Lemeshow (2000). *Applied logistic regression.* New York, Wiley & Sons.

Jugendministerkonferenz (2004). „*Gemeinsamer Rahmen der Länder für die frühe Bildung in Kindertageseinrichtungen – Beschluss der Jugendministerkonferenz (13.-14.05.2004), Beschluss der Kultusministerkonferenz (03.–04.06.2004)."* http://www.bildungsserver.de/db/mlesen. html?Id= 25908. (Stand 21.11.2017).

Jungbauer, J. and S. Ehlen (2015). *"Stress and Burnout Risk in Nursery School Teachers: Results from a Survey"*. *Gesundheitswesen 77(6): 418-423*.

Klein, J., K. Grosse Frie, K. Blum, J. Siegrist and O. dem Knesebeck (2010). *"Effort-reward imbalance, job strain and burnout among clinicians in surgery."* *Psychother Psychosom Med Psychol 60(9-10): 374-379*.

Koch, P., J. F. Kersten, J. Stranzinger and A. Nienhaus (2017). *"The effect of effort-reward imbalance on the health of childcare workers in Hamburg: a longitudinal study"*. *Journal of Occupational Medicine and Toxicology 12(1): 16*.

Koch, P., A. Schablon, U. Latza and A. Nienhaus (2014). *"Musculoskeletal pain and effort-reward imbalance - a systematic review"*. *BMC Public Health 14: 37*.

Koch, P., J. Stranzinger, A. Nienhaus and A. Kozak (2015). *"Musculoskeletal Symptoms and Risk of Burnout in Child Care Workers - A Cross-Sectional Study"*. *PLoSOne 10(10): e0140980*.

Kraatz, S., J. Lang, T. Kraus, E. Munster and E. Ochsmann (2013). *"The incremental effect of psychosocial workplace factors on the development of neck and shoulder disorders: a systematic review of longitudinal studies"*. *Int Arch Occup Environ Health 86(4): 375-395*.

Krause-Girth, C. (2011). *„Geschlechtsspezifische Prävention psychosozialer Probleme in städtischen Kindertagesstätten und ihre Auswirkungen auf die Arbeitsbelastung und Gesundheit des pädagogischen Personals 2008–2010"*. Für die Hans-Böckler-Stiftung. https://www.boeckler.de/pdf_fof/96813.pdf. (Stand 20.11.2017).

Krause, N., B. Burgel and D. Rempel (2010). *"Effort-reward imbalance and one-year change in neck-shoulder and upper extremity pain among call center computer operators"*.Scand J Work Environ Health 36(1): 42-53.

Lang, J., E. Ochsmann, T. Kraus and J. W. Lang (2012). *"Psychosocial work stressors as antecedents of musculoskeletal problems: a systematic review and meta-analysis of stability-adjusted longitudinal studies."* *Soc Sci Med 75(7): 1163-1174*.

Lapointe, J., C. E. Dionne, C. Brisson and S. Montreuil (2013). *"Effort-reward imbalance and video display unit postural risk factors interact in women on the incidence of musculoskeletal symptoms"*. *Work 44(2): 133-143*.

Lau, B. (2008). *"Effort-reward imbalance and overcommitment in employees in a Norwegian municipality: a cross sectional study"*. *J Occup Med Toxicol 3:9*.

LärmVibrationsArbSchV (2007). *„Verordnung zum Schutz der Beschäftigten vor Gefährdungen durch Lärm und Vibrationen (Lärm- und Vibrations-Arbeitsschutzverordnung)"*. http://www.gesetze-im-internet.de/l_rmvibrationsarbschv/ (Stand 21.11.2017).

Limm, H., H. Gündel, M. Heinmüller, B. Marten-Mittag, U. M. Nater, J. Siegrist and P. Angerer (2011). *"Stress management interventions in the workplace improve stress reactivity: a randomised controlled trial"*. *Occup Environ Med. 2011 Feb;68(2):126-33*.

Loerbroks, A., H. Meng, M. L. Chen, R. Herr, P. Angerer and J. Li (2014). *"Primary school teachers in China: associations of organizational justice and effort-reward imbalance with burnout and intentions to leave the profession in a cross-sectional sample"*. *Int Arch Occup Environ Health 87(7): 695-703*.

Losch, D. (2016). *„Lärm als Stressor in der Kindertagesstätte"*. *Zentralblatt für Arbeitsmedizin, Arbeitsschutz und Ergonomie 66(1): 20-28*.

Lundberg, U. (1999). *"Stress Responses in Low Status Jobs and Their Relationship to Health Risks: Musculoskeletal Disorders"*. *Annals of the New York Academy of Sciences 896(1): 162-172*.

McGrath, B. J. (2007). *"Identifying health and safety risks for childcare workers"*. *AAOHN journal 55(8): 321-325*.

Neitzel, R. L., E. B. Svensson, S. K. Sayler and J. Ann-Christin (2014). *"A comparison of occupational and nonoccupational noise exposures in Sweden"*. *Noise Health 16(72): 270-278*.

Nübling, M. (2015). *Personal Communication. Freiburg.*

Nübling, M., A. Seidler, S. Garthus-Niegel, U. Latza, M. Wagner, J. Hegewald, F. Liebers, S. Jankowiak, I. Zwiener, P. S. Wild and S. Letzel (2013). *"The Gutenberg Health Study: measuring psychosocial factors at work and predicting health and work-related outcomes with the ERI and the COPSOQ questionnaire".BMC Public Health 13: 538.*

Paulsen, R. (2004). *"Noise Exposure in Kindergartens". 30.Jahrestagung für Akustik – Europäische Akustik-Ausstellung. http://www.conforg.fr/cfadaga2004/cdrom/data/procs/articles/000256.pdf (Stand 20.11.2017).*

Podsakoff, P. M., S. B. MacKenzie, J. Y. Lee and N. P. Podsakoff (2003). *"Common method biases i behavioral research: a critical review of the literature and recommended remedies". J Appl Psychol 88(5): 879-903.*

Rudow, B. (2004). *„Belastungen im Erzieher/innenberuf". Bildung & Wissenschaft(6): 6-11.*

Rudow, B. (2005). *„Arbeits-und Gesundheitsschutz bei Erzieherinnen in Sachsen-Anhalt". Forschungsbericht im Auftrag der Unfallkasse Sachsen-Anhalt. Merseburg & Viernheim.*

Rudow, B. (2015). *„Belastungen von Erzieherinnen in der Arbeit an der Schule (Berliner Modellprojekt) – BEAS Berlin". Zusammenfassung des Projektberichts, Gewerkschaft für Erziehung und Wissenschaft, Berlin.*

Rugulies, R. and N. Krause (2008). *"Effort-reward imbalance and incidence of low back and neck injuries in San Francisco transit operators". Occup Environ Med 65(8): 525-533.*

Scharf, T. and D. Groneberg (2015). *Lärm in deutschen Kindertageseinrichtungen: Eine Pilotstudie mit praktischer Handlungsanweisung zu lärmreduzierenden Maßnahmen. RiRe-Risiken und Ressourcen in Gesundheitsdienst und Wohlfahrtspflege. A. Nienhaus. Landsberg am Lech, Ecomed Medizin. 2: 75-82.*

Schaufeli, W. B. and B. P. Buunk (2003). *Burnout: An overview of 25 years of research and theorizing. The handbook of work and health psychology. M. J. Schabracq, J. A. Winnubst and C. L. Cooper. New York, Wiley & Sons: 383-425.*

Scheuch, K. and R. Seibt (2007). *Arbeits- und persönlichkeitsbedingte Beziehungen zu Burnout – eine kritische Betrachtung. Arbeit und Gesundheit. P. G. Richter, R. Rau and S. Mühlpfordt. Lengerich, Pabst Science Publishers: 42-54.*

Schreyer, I., M. Krause, M. Brandl and O. Nicko (2014). *AQUA Arbeitsplatz und Qualität in Kitas Ergebnisse einer bundesweiten Befragung. München, Staatsinstitut für Frühpädagogik.*

Seibt, R., J. Malbrich and D. Dutschke (2006). *„Zusammenhänge von Einflussfaktoren und Burnout-Risiko bei Lehrern und Erziehern". Das Gesundheitswesen 68(07): A116.*

Seti, C. L. (2008). *"Causes and treatment of burnout in residential child care workers: A review of the research". Residential Treatment for Children & Youth 24(3): 197-229.*

SGB VIII (2008). *Sozialgesetzbuch-Achtes Buch – Kinder- und Jugendhilfe Artikel 1 §24 Anspruch auf Förderung in Tageseinrichtungen und in der Kindertagespflege. https://www.bgbl.de/xaver/ bgbl/start.xav#__bgbl__%2F%2F*%5B%40attr_id%3D%27bgbl108s2403.pdf%27%5D__ 1511252790968 (Stand 21.11.2017).*

Siegrist, J. (1996). *"Adverse health effects of high-effort/low-reward conditions". J Occup Health Psychol 1(1): 27-41.*

Siegrist, J. and N. Dragano (2008). *„Psychosoziale Belastungen und Erkrankungsrisiken im Erwerbsleben". Bundesgesundheitsblatt-Gesundheitsforschung-Gesundheitsschutz 51(3): 305-312.*

Siegrist, J., D. Starke, T. Chandola, I. Godin, M. Marmot, I. Niedhammer and R. Peter (2004). *"The measurement of effort-reward imbalance at work: European comparisons". Soc Sci Med 58(8): 1483-1499.*

Simon, M., P. Tackenberg, A. Nienhaus, M. Estryn-Behar, P. M. Conway and H. M. Hasselhorn (2008). *"Back or neck-pain-related disability of nursing staff in hospitals, nursing homes and home care in seven countries--results from the European NEXT-Study". Int J Nurs Stud 45(1): 24-34.*

Sinn-Behrendt, A., L. Sica, V. Bopp, R. Bruder, M. Brehmen, D. Groneberg, E.-M. Burford, P. Schreiber, B. Weber and R. Ellegast (2015). *Projekt ErgoKiTa – Prävention von Muskel-Skelett-Belastungen bei Erzieherinnen und Erziehern in Kindertageseinrichtungen. Deutsche Gesetzliche Unfallversicherung (DGUV). Berlin.*

Sjodin, F., A. Kjellberg, A. Knutsson, U. Landstrom and L. Lindberg (2012). *"Noise and stress effects on preschool personnel". Noise Health 14(59): 166-178.*

Sjodin, F., A. Kjellberg, A. Knutsson, U. Landstrom and L. Lindberg (2014). *"Measures against preschool noise and its adverse effects on the personnel: an intervention study". Int Arch Occup Environ Healt 87(1): 95-110.*

Spence Laschinger, H. K. and J. Finegan (2008). *"Situational and dispositional predictors of nurse manager burnout: a time-lagged analysis". J Nurs Manag 16(5): 601-607.*

Spieß, C. K. and F. G. Westermaier (2016). *„Berufsgruppe Erzieherin: zufrieden mit der Arbeit, aber nicht mit der Entlohnung". DIW-Wochenbericht 83(43): 1023-1033.*

Statistisches Bundesamt (2016). *Kinder und tätige Personen in Tageseinrichtungen und in öffentlicher Kindertagespflege am 01.03.2016. Statiken der Kinder- und Jugendhilfe. Wiesbaden, Statistisches Bundesamt.*

Theorell, T. (1999). *"How to deal with stress in organizations? – a health perspective on theory and practice". Scandinavian Journal of Work, Environment & Health: 616-624.*

Thinschmidt, M. (2010). *„Belastungen am Arbeitsplatz Kindertagesstätte – Übersicht zu zentralen Ergebnissen aus vorliegenden Studien". Ratgeber. Betriebliche Gesundheitsförderung im Sozial-und Erziehungsdienst: 17-26.*

Truchnon-Gagnon, C. H., R. (1988). *"Noise in Day-Care Centers for Chlidren". Noise Control Engineerin Journal 30(2): 57-64.*

ver.di (2014). Vereinte Dienstleistungsgewerkschaft: *„ver.di Tarifkonferenz fordert Aufwertung für den Sozial- und Erziehungsdienst". https://stuttgart.verdi.de/branchen/gemeinden/++co++edb08 e24-7558-11e4-9886-525400a933ef (Stand 20.11.2017).*

Verbeek, J. H., E. Kateman, T. C. Morata, W. A. Dreschler and C. Mischke (2014). *"Interventions to prevent occupational noise-induced hearing loss: a Cochrane systematic review". Int J Audiol 53 Suppl 2: S84-96.*

Viernickel, S., I. Nentwig-Gesemann, K. Nicolai, S. Schwarz and L. Zenker (2013). *Schlüssel zu guter Bildung, Erziehung und Betreuung: Bildungsaufgaben, Zeitkontingente und strukturelle Rahmenbedingungen in Kindertageseinrichtungen, Der Paritätische Gesamtverband.*

Viernickel, S., A. Voss, E. Mauz, F. Gerstenberg and M. Schumann (2013). *STEGE – Strukturqualität und Erzieher_innengesundheit in Kindertageseinrichtungen. Wissenschaftlicher Abschlussbericht. http://www.gew.de/index.php?eID=dumpFile&t=f&f=20674&token=9d0413d1612a043e64cd-74e9e71d51fccefd13ec&sdownload= (Stand 21.11.2017).*

von dem Knesebeck, O., K. David and J. Siegrist (2005). *"[Psychosocial stress at work and musculoskeletal pain among police officers in special forces]". Das Gesundheitswesen 67(8-9): 674-679.*

Wang, Y., A. Ramos, H. Wu, L. Liu, X. Yang, J. Wang and L. Wang (2015). *"Relationship between occupational stress and burnout among Chinese teachers: a cross-sectional survey in Liaoning, China". Int Arch Occup Environ Health 88(5): 589-597.*

Weyers, S., R. Peter, H. Boggild, H. J. Jeppesen and J. Siegrist (2006). *"Psychosocial work stress is associated with poor self-rated health in Danish nurses: a test of the effort-reward imbalance model". Scand J Caring Sci 20(1): 26-34.*

4 Abkürzungsverzeichnis

BGW	Berufsgenossenschaft für Gesundheitsdienst und Wohlfahrtspflege
CI	Confidence Interval
COPSOQ	Copenhagen Psychosocial Questionnaire
ERI	Effort-Reward-Imbalance
Kita	Kindertagesstätte
MSB	Muskuloskelettale Beschwerden
OR	Odds Ratio
OVC	Overcommitment
RCT	Randomized Controlled Trial
SD	Standard Deviation
SOEP	Sozio-oekonomisches Panel
TOP	Technisch-organisatorisch-personenbezogen

5 Abbildungsverzeichnis

6 Tabellenverzeichnis